CAWSON

ORAL PATHOLOGY
PBK ED

Churchill Livingstone
EDINBURGH LONDON MELBOURNE AND NEW YORK 1987

1 | Developmental Defects of Teeth

Aetiology

Genetic
Amelogenesis imperfecta—hypoplastic or hypocalcified types.
Dentinogenesis imperfecta.

Acquired
Rickets.
Severe metabolic disturbances.
Fluorosis.
Tetracycline pigmentation.

Microscopy

Amelogenesis imperfecta hypoplastic type. Defective matrix formation—enamel irregular, overall thin, sometimes nodular or pitted. Well-calcified, hard, translucent.
Hypocalcified type. Normal matrix formation and morphology but soft and chalky.
Dentinogenesis imperfecta. Mantle (superficial) dentine, regular tubules; remainder—a few irregular tubules, inclusion of small blood vessels, and enamel defects also.
Severe metabolic disturbances. Typically affect enamel matrix producing linear pitting enamel defects corresponding to degree of tooth formation at time of illness.
Tetracycline pigmentation. Teeth usually of normal form but stained yellow, degrading to grey or brown. Hard sections show yellow fluorescence along incremental lines under UV light.

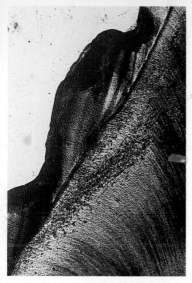

Fig. 1 Amelogenesis imperfecta: hypoplastic type.

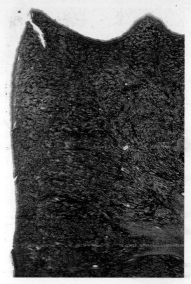

Fig. 2 Dentinogenesis imperfecta.

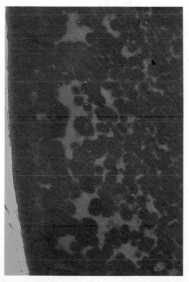

Fig. 3 Rickets.

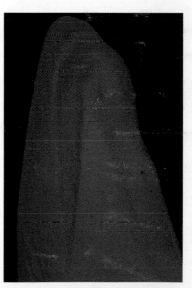

Fig. 4 Tetracycline pigmentation.

2 | Dental Caries (1)

1. Bacteria—probably mainly acidogenic and glucan-forming strains of *Strep. mutans*. Other viridans streptococci, lactobacilli or actinomyces may contribute, possibly at different stages.
2. Plaque. Adherent meshwork of bacteria in polysaccharides, thickest in stagnation areas, concentrates bacterial acid production and delays buffering by saliva.
3. Susceptible tooth surface and (possibly) immune responses.
4. Frequent supply of bacterial substrate—mainly sugar (sucrose).

Enamel caries

Pre-invasive stage (submicroscopic)—bacterial acid leads to production of increasing size and numbers of submicroscopic pores in enamel. Light microscopy shows conical area of change with apex deeply, comprising
a. dense surface zone (more radiopaque) with enhanced striae of Retzius
b. main body of lesion
c. dark zone
d. peripheral translucent zone.
Degrees of demineralisation in different zones assessed by polarised light studies and microradiography. Progressive demineralisation eventually allows entry to bacteria.
Secondary enamel caries. Bacteria reach and spread along the amelodentinal junction and attack enamel from beneath over a wide area.

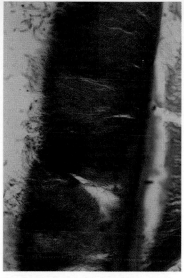

Fig. 5 Bacterial plaque on enamel surface.

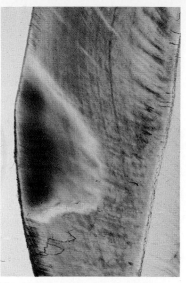

Fig. 6 Early caries (pre-invasive stage).

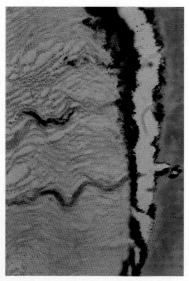

Fig. 7 Secondary enamel caries.

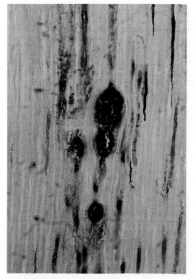

Fig. 8 Caries of dentine.

Dental Caries (2)

Dentine caries

Dentine is demineralised by bacterial acids from bacteria spreading along amelodentinal junction and invaded via the tubules, a conical lesion being formed.
Walls of tubules in softened dentine become distended by bacteria. Intervening dentine breaks down to form liquefaction foci and the tissue progressively disintegrates.

Dentinal reactions

Dead tracts
Odontoblasts are killed in acute caries and pulpal ends of tubules sealed off by calcified material.

Translucent zones
In very chronic caries or attrition, tubule walls become progressively calcified (peritubular dentine) until tubules are obliterated.

Secondary (reparative) dentine
Regular tubulated dentine forms under chronic lesions. Irregular dentine with few, irregular tubules forms beneath more acute lesions.

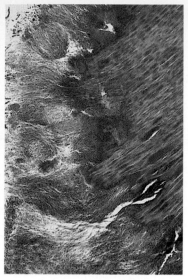

Fig. 9 Plaque invading dentine.

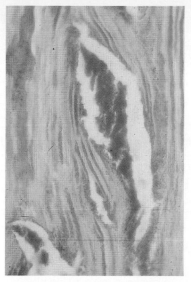

Fig. 10 Bacteria destroying dentine. (High power.)

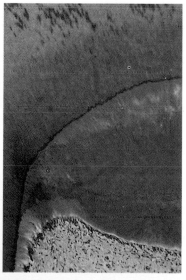

Fig. 11 Secondary (reactionary) dentine.

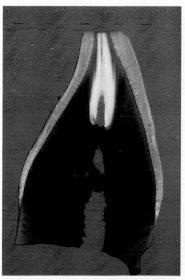

Fig. 12 Translucent zone (attrition).

Aetiology

1. Caries (most commonly).
2. Traumatic exposure (cavity preparation fracture or cracked tooth syndrome).
3. Thermal or chemical irritation from fillings.

Closed pulpitis

Acute closed pulpitis

Pathology

All degrees of severity, namely
a. acute hyperaemia and oedema
b. progressive infiltration by neutrophils
c. destruction of specialised pulp cells
d. abscess formation
e. cellulitis
f. necrosis.
(Little correlation between symptoms and histological picture but acute pulp pain usually indicative of irreversibly severe pulpitis.)

Chronic closed pulpitis

Pathology

a. Predominantly mononuclear inflammatory cells (lymphocytes, plasma cells and macrophages).
b. Initially localised pulp damage. Destruction of pulp often relatively slow.
c. Often an incomplete calcific barrier around inflammatory focus.
d. Usually, necrosis of pulp eventually results.

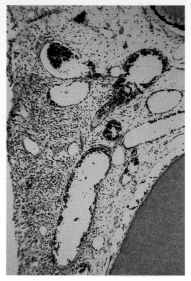

Fig. 13 Hyperaemia of pulp.

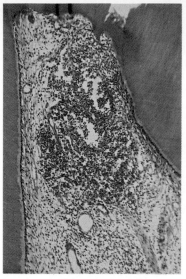

Fig. 14 Localised pulp abscess.

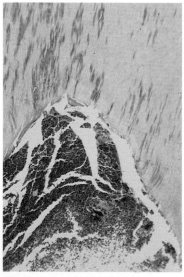

Fig. 15 Advanced pulp abscess.

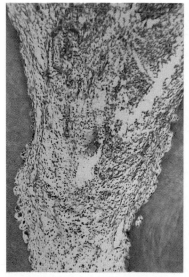

Fig. 16 Cellulitis of pulp.

Open pulpitis

Acute open pulpitis
Rapidly progressive acute inflammation secondary to acute exposure of pulp.

Chronic open pulpitis
Carious destruction of crown of tooth but survival of pulp (uncommon).
Pulp replaced by granulation tissue which gradually proliferates through exposure.
Granulation tissue acquires epithelial covering and inflammatory changes subside. Progressive fibrosis produces a pulp polyp.

Other pulp changes

a. Calcification.
   (i) Secondary to pulpitis (see above).
   (ii) Pulp stones. Rounded masses of ectopic dentine formation. Chance finding on radiographs or on histology.
   (iii) Diffuse calcification. Fine granular deposits fusing to form larger irregular masses.
b. Internal resorption (see p. 13).

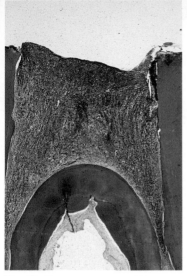

Fig. 17 Chronic open pulpitis.

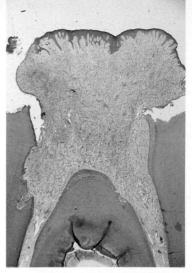

Fig. 18 Open pulpitis; epithelialised polyp.

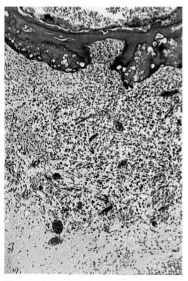

Fig. 19 Calcification ('dentine bridge') under pulpitis.

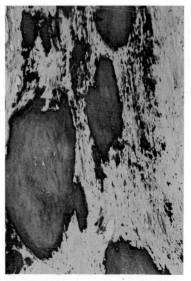

Fig. 20 Pulp stones and calcifications.

4 | Apical Periodontitis

Aetiology

1. Secondary to caries and pulp necrosis in most cases).
2. Trauma to tooth severing apical vessels.
3. Root canal treatment (irritant medicaments or overextension).

Pathology

Acute. Accumulation of acute inflammatory cells (neutrophils) and fluid exudate in potential space between apex and periapical bone. If neglected, suppuration and resorption, usually of buccal plate of bone. Sinus formation on gum overlying apex of tooth. In deciduous molars, inflammation often interradicular, i.e. overlying permanent successor.

Chronic. Low grade inflammation. Proliferation of granulation tissue (fibroblasts and capillary loops). Varying density of inflammatory infiltrate. Formation of rounded nodule of granulation tissue (apical granuloma) with resorption of periapical bone to accommodate it.

Epithelial content. Rests of Malassez often destroyed by inflammation. If not, they may proliferate in apical granulomas to form microcysts. Epithelial lining variable in thickness. Eventually, a periodontal cyst may thus form.

Pus formation. Neutrophil infiltration and low grade suppuration usually leading eventually to discharge via sinus on gum or occasionally on skin over apex.

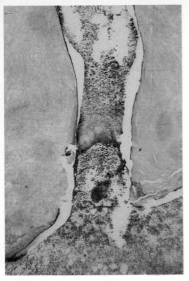

Fig. 21 Acute periapical periodontitis.

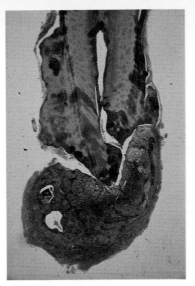

Fig. 22 Apical granuloma.

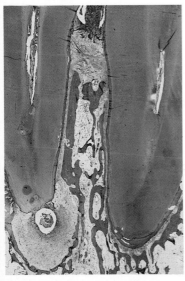

Fig. 23 Apical granuloma in situ.

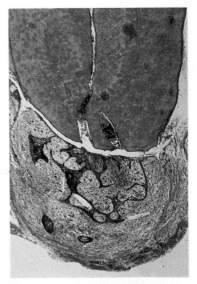

Fig. 24 Apical granuloma with epithelial proliferation.

5 | Resorption

Aetiology

Normal in deciduous teeth before shedding.
Pathological
1. Idiopathic. Internal or external.
2. Secondary (local inflammation, pressure from malposed tooth or tumour, orthodontic movement, replantation, buried teeth).

Pathology

Idiopathic. Progressive giant cell resorption, mainly of dentine. Sometimes intermittent reparative activity to form complex pattern of resorption and bone-like reparative tissue. Resorption (internal or external) can expose pulp. Pulpitis follows.
Secondary. Usually localised giant cell activity. Variable reparative activity with hard tissue deposition.

6 | Hypercementosis

Aetiology

Ageing; chronic apical periodontitis (adjacent to resorption); buried teeth, Paget's disease; cementomas (p. 49–51).

Pathology

Usually lamellar—sequential deposition of layers of cementum forming smooth thickening of root. Rarely (Paget's disease or cementoblastoma) irregular jigsaw-puzzle ('mosaic') pattern of intermittent deposition and resorption.

ORAL PATHOLOGY

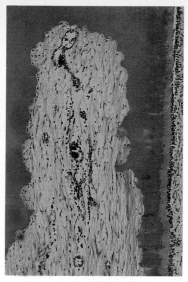

Fig. 25 Internal resorption of dentine.

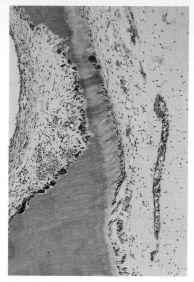

Fig. 26 External resorption.

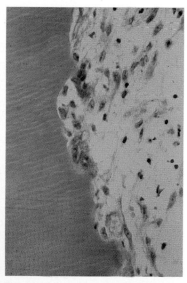

Fig. 27 Internal resorption showing giant cells.

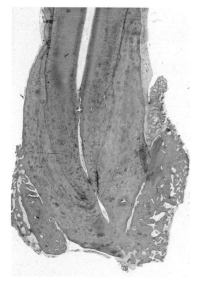

Fig. 28 Hypercementosis—lamellar and irregular.

Acute ulcerative gingivitis

Aetiology

Otherwise healthy young adults affected. Aetiology unknown but associated with
a. poor oral hygiene
b. smoking
c. upper respiratory tract infections
d. stress.

Microbiology

Overwhelming proliferation of Gram-negative anaerobic bacteria traditionally termed *Fusobacterium nucleatum* and *Borrelia (Treponema) vincenti*. Other anaerobes may also be involved.
Smear shows fusospirochaetal complex and polymorphs.

Pathology

Gingival necrosis and non-specific ulceration covered by slough containing fusiforms and spirochaetes. Tissue invasion by spirochaetes. Progressive destruction of marginal gingivae and then of deeper supporting tissues. No generalised stomatitis.

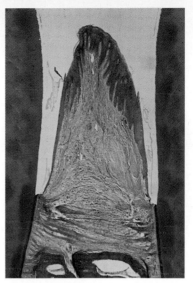

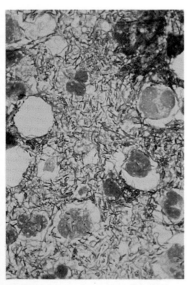

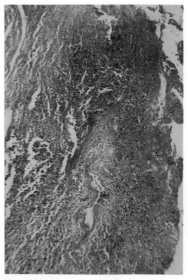

Fig. 29 Normal human adult buccal gingiva.

Fig. 30 Normal human adult interdental gingiva.

Fig. 31 Acute ulcerative gingivitis; fusobacterial complex in smear.

Fig. 32 Acute ulcerative gingivitis: gingival necrosis.

Chronic gingivitis

Aetiology

Accumulation of plaque in gingival sulcus. Mixed non-specific bacterial complex, initially Gram-positive and aerobic, but becoming gradually more Gram-negative and anaerobic.

Microscopy

There is plaque attached to the tooth surface. Filamentous bacteria appear predominant but their role is unknown.

Inflammation is sharply restricted to the vicinity of the plaque. Variable degrees of hyperaemia are seen. The inflammatory infiltrate is predominantly mononuclear (lymphocytes and plasma cells). Epithelial attachment extends to the amelocemental junction and (by definition) there is no destruction of supporting tissues.

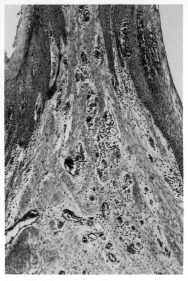

Fig. 33 Marginal gingivitis, early hyperaemic stage.

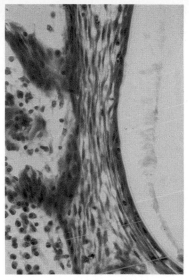

Fig. 34 Junctional epithelium and epithelial attachment on enamel.

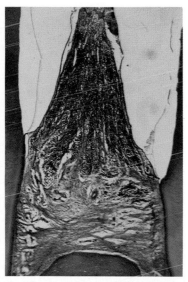

Fig. 35 Marginal gingivitis: dense chronic inflammatory infiltrate.

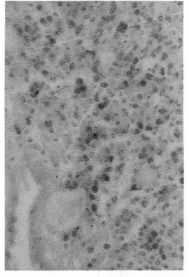

Fig. 36 Immunoperoxidase showing antibody production in plasma cells.

Chronic periodontitis

Aetiology

Persistence of bacterial plaque. Progression of inflammation, with tissue destruction a common but not invariable sequel to chronic gingivitis; wide individual variation for unknown reasons.

Microbiology and immunology

Many potent pathogens (e.g. *Bacteroides* species, *Capnocytophaga*, *Clostridia*, *Fusobacteria*, etc.) isolated from periodontal pockets, but individual role in tissue destruction uncertain. Some (e.g. *Actinomyces* species) produce bone resorbing factors. Defensive immune response (antibody production and cellular immunity) to plaque bacteria detectable. Evidence of immunologically mediated tissue destruction speculative only and not consistent with histological findings. Periodontal destruction accelerated in immunodeficient patients but host factors affecting prognosis of periodontal disease not identified in otherwise healthy persons.

Microscopy

1. Plaque and often calculus on tooth surface extending into pockets.
2. Inflammation (predominantly mononuclear infiltrate) of gingival margins and pocket walls. Inflammation typically limited to vicinity of plaque and remaining well clear of alveolar bone crest or most superficial periodontal ligament fibres.
3. Loss of periodontal ligament fibres.
4. Destruction of alveolar bone but osteoclasts rarely seen.
5. Formation of epithelium-lined pockets with epithelial attachment as the floor.
6. Gradual rootward progression of these changes. Eventual loosening of teeth.
Tissue destruction usually uniform along arch (horizontal bone loss); less often, accelerated localised destruction of bone around individual teeth (vertical bone loss). Occasionally more rapid destruction of periodontal ligament than alveolar bone with extension of pocketing between tooth and bone (infra-bony pocketing).

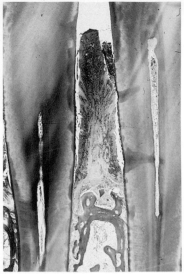

Fig. 37 Advanced chronic periodontitis. Note inflammatory infiltrate localised to vicinity of plaque.

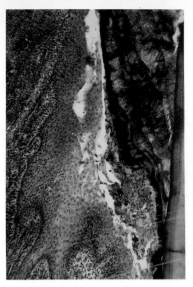

Fig. 38 Periodontal pocket: plaque and calculus, and epithelial lining.

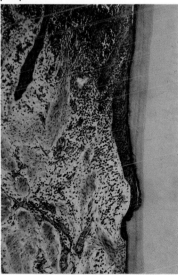

Fig. 39 Migration of epithelial attachment along cementum.

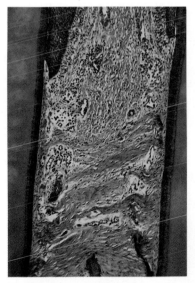

Fig. 40 Chronic periodontitis. Inflammation-free zone between floor of pocket and bony crest.

Periodontal (lateral abscess)

Aetiology

Usually a complication of advanced periodontitis. May be due to injury to pocket floor (?food-packing) or more virulent infection.

Pathology

Rapid acceleration of periodontal destruction.
Destruction of epithelial pocket lining.
Dense neutrophil infiltrate and suppuration.
Widespread osteoclastic resorption of bone increasing width and depth of pocket to form deep infrabony pocket.
Pus may exude from pocket mouth or point on attached gingiva.

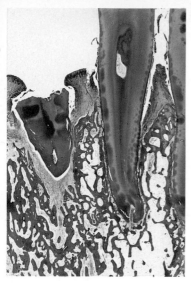

Fig. 41 Late periodontitis with infra-bony pocket.

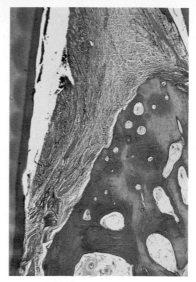

Fig. 42 Higher power view of infra-bony pocket.

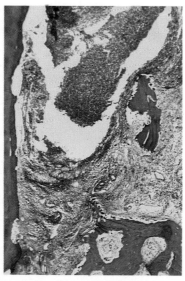

Fig. 43 Periodontal abscess.

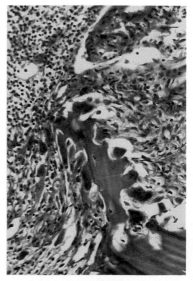

Fig. 44 Giant cells resorbing bony floor of periodontal abscess.

Gingival recession

Aetiology

Wear and tear ('senile') from over-vigorous toothbrushing. Severe uncontrolled ulcerative gingivitis. Some cases of chronic periodontitis.

Microscopy

Gradual destruction of gingival tissue, periodontal ligament and bone, all at similar rates. No pocket formed. Low grade minimal chronic inflammation.

Gingival swelling

Microscopy

Acute (myelomonocytic) leukaemia
Exaggerated response to plaque, with gross infiltration of gingivae by leukaemic cells, gingival swelling, and accelerated periodontal destruction.

Fibrous hyperplasia
Hereditary type. Generalised smooth gingival swelling may overgrow and conceal erupting teeth.
Drug-associated hyperplasia produces bulbous swellings of interdental papillae. Both show hyperplasia of gingival collagen with 'stretching' of elongated rete ridges.

Pathology

Pregnancy epulis (pregnancy tumour)
Dilated thin-walled vessels in loose oedematous connective tissue. Superimposed inflammation often produces same appearance as pyogenic granuloma.

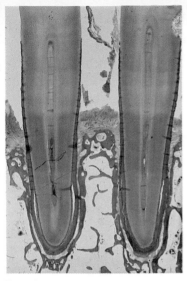

Fig. 45 Gingival and periodontal recession.

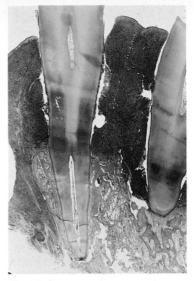

Fig. 46 Acute myelomonocytic leukaemia—gingival infiltration.

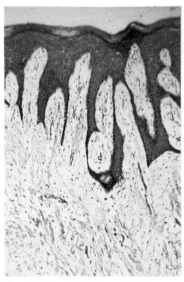

Fig. 47 Gingival fibromatosis.

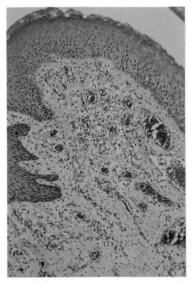

Fig. 48 Pregnancy epulis.

Periodontal (radicular) cysts

Aetiology

Pulp death, apical periodontitis, proliferation of epithelial rests of Malassez, cystic change in epithelium. Expansion of cyst by hydrostatic pressure. Resorption of surrounding bone.

Incidence

65%–70% of jaw cysts. Most common cause of chronic swellings of the jaws.

Pathology

Early. Variable thickness of squamous epithelial lining, often in arcaded pattern, sometimes destroyed in part by inflammation. Fibrous cyst wall with chronic inflammatory infiltrate. Plasma cells are numerous and sometimes predominant.
Late. The epithelium is usually thin and the inflammatory infiltrate minimal.

Residual cysts
The causative tooth is extracted, leaving a residual cyst. They are, typically found late, and show late-type features.

Lateral cysts
These are found in the periodontal ligament beside a tooth related to lateral branch of the root canal of a dead tooth.

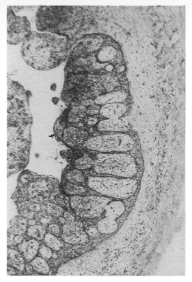

Fig. 49 Arcaded epithelium of cyst lining.

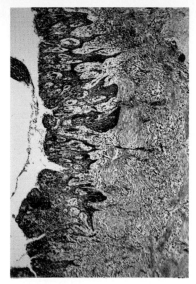

Fig. 50 Inflamed cyst with irregular epithelial lining.

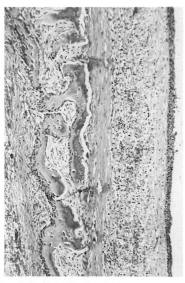

Fig. 51 Complete epithelial, fibrous and bony cyst wall.

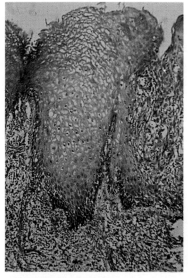

Fig. 52 Thick epithelium lining periodontal cyst.

Periodontal (radicular) cysts (cont)

Clefts
Cholesterol from breakdown of blood cells forms needle-like clefts in giant cells, associated with deposits of blood pigments in walls of cysts. Clefts are often also seen in cyst contents.

Hyaline bodies
Hyaline (Rushton) bodies are thin refractile rod-like or hair-pin or other shapes. Staining is variable. Their nature is unknown. They are possibly an epithelial product or haematogenous in origin.

Goblet cells
Mucous cell metaplasia can produce mucin-filled goblet cells in epithelial cyst lining.

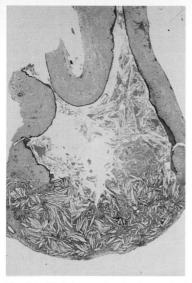

Fig. 53 Cleft formation in the wall of a cyst.

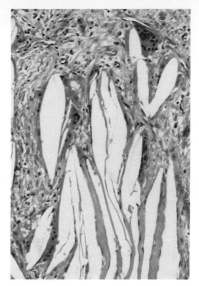

Fig. 54 Clefts with giant cells and deposits of haemosiderin.

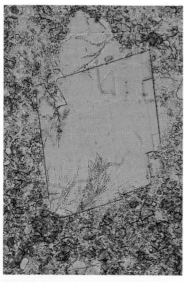

Fig. 55 Cholesterol crystal from cyst fluid.

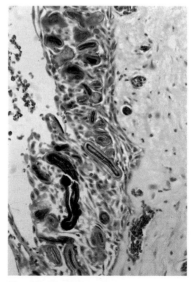

Fig. 56 Hyaline bodies in cyst wall.

Cysts of the Jaws (3)

Dentigerous cysts

Aetiology

Cystic change in remains of enamel organ after completion of enamel formation. Developmental defect of unknown cause.

Incidence

15–18% of jaw cysts. Male to female ratio more than 2 to 1.

Microscopy

Cyst wall attached to neck of tooth at or near amelocemental junction.
Lining of cyst (probably originating from external enamel epithelium) typically appears as a thin flat layer of squamous cells without defined layer of basal cells. Inner enamel epithelium covering crown of teeth usually lost. Fibrous wall typically without inflammatory infiltrate, unless secondarily infected.
Mucous cells relatively common.

Eruption cysts
Strictly, a soft tissue cyst in the gingiva overlying unerupted tooth. Probably a superficial dentigerous cyst.

Microscopy

Thin fibrous wall with thin squamous epithelial lining deeply and oral mucosal epithelium superficially. Variable inflammatory infiltrate in the wall.

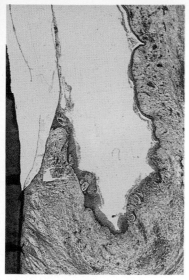

Fig. 57 Dentigerous cyst with enamel epithelium between enamel space (left) and cyst (right).

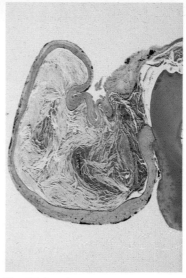

Fig. 58 Dentigerous cyst showing attachment at neck of tooth.

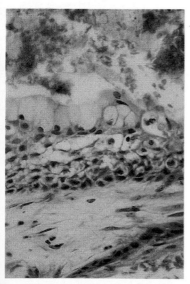

Fig. 59 Goblet cells in dentigerous cyst lining.

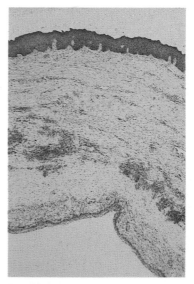

Fig. 60 Eruption cyst with mucosa overlying cyst wall.

Primordial cyst (odontogenic keratocyst)

Aetiology

Unknown. Presumably originates in primordial odontogenic epithelium (any part of dental lamina or remnants thereof) or enamel organ before start of amelogenesis; tooth sometimes missing.

Incidence

About 10% of odontogenic cysts. Male to female ratio about 1.5 to 1. Most frequent in young adults or at age 50–60; possibly then as a result of slow growth and late detection.

Pathology

About 75% in body or ramus of mandible. Typically, infiltrative growth into cancellous bone forming extensive pseudoloculated area of radiolucency with little expansion of bone.

Microscopy

Characteristic lining of epithelium of even thickness, 5–8 cells thick, and flat basement membrane. Tall, palisaded basal cell layer and thin eosinophilic layer of prekeratin. Orthokeratinisation in minority (about 30%) occasionally with keratin forming semisolid cyst contents.
Epithelium typically much folded and tends to separate from fibrous wall. Occasionally daughter cysts or islands of odontogenic epithelium in wall. Inflammatory infiltrate typically absent but infection and inflammation causes lining to resemble that of periodontal cyst.
Strong tendency to recur.

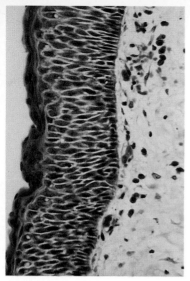

Fig. 61 Typical primordial cyst lining.

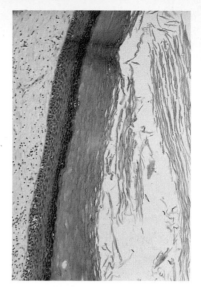

Fig. 62 Primordial cyst with keratinisation.

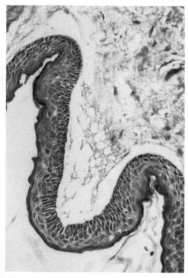

Fig. 63 Primordial cyst. Loose attachment of lining to fibrous wall.

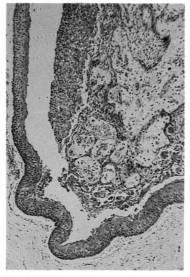

Fig. 64 Primordial cyst with part of wall inflamed.

Nasopalatine (incisive canal; median palatine) cyst

Aetiology
Proliferation of epithelial remnants of lining of nasopalatine duct.

Microscopy
Midline cyst of anterior maxilla.
Lining of squamous and/or ciliated columnar epithelium.
Characteristically, a neurovascular bundle (also from incisive canal) and sometimes salivary acini may be found in cyst wall.

Globulomaxillary cyst

Aetiology
Unknown—possibly several entities including periodontal cysts but so rare that consensus impossible.

Pathology
By definition forms in anterior maxilla between lateral incisor and canine, both of which are vital, but these criteria often not completely fulfiled. Fibrous wall lining may be squamous, columnar or columnar ciliated epithelium.

Nasolabial cyst

Aetiology
Unknown.
Exceedingly rare soft tissue cyst external to alveolar ridge beneath ala nasi. Aetiology unknown but possibly arises from remnants of lower end of nasolacrimal duct. Seen at almost any age but peak incidence at 40–50.

Microscopy
Lining classically (but often not) of non-ciliated columnar epithelium but may be squamous or ciliated with fibrous wall.

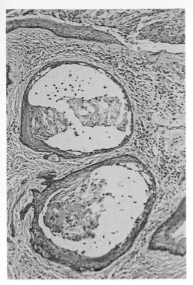

Fig. 65 Daughter cysts in primordial cyst wall.

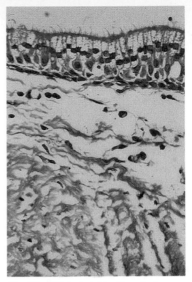

Fig. 66 Ciliated epithelium lining nasopalatine cyst.

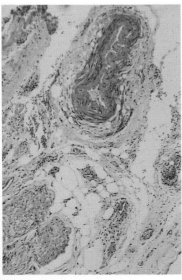

Fig. 67 Neurovascular bundle in nasopalatine cyst wall.

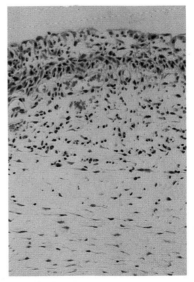

Fig. 68 Nasolabial cyst.

Cysts within tumours

Cysts within tumours can be mistaken for simple cysts clinically and radiographically but precise nature confirmed by microscopy. Most common in ameloblastoma.
Calcifying odontogenic cyst can be a cyst or solid tumour.

Microscopy

Cystic ameloblastoma
Extensive cystic change (see p. 42) can overgrow the tumour. Lining becomes flattened and may be indistinguishable from simple cyst in part. Elsewhere ameloblastoma cells more obvious in cyst lining and typical tumour forms mural thickening.

Calcifying odontogenic cyst

Though often cystic, this lesion can also be solid and may be a benign odontogenic tumour.

Incidence

Rare. Any age affected but most often detected in second decade.

Microscopy

Fibrous wall. Lining predominantly of squamous epithelium but basal layer may be columnar and ameloblast-like. Abnormal keratinisation of spinous cells produces ghost cells consisting of distended eosinophilic epithelial cells either anuclear or occasionally containing nuclear remnants. Patchy calcification may develop in them. Associated or induced odontogenic tumors or hamartomas not infrequent adjacently in fibrous wall.

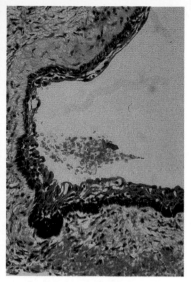

Fig. 69 Cyst in ameloblastoma.

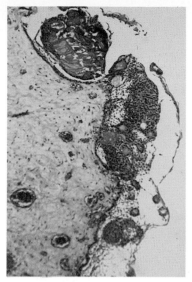

Fig. 70 Calcifying odontogenic cyst with ghost cells.

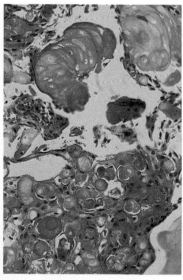

Fig. 71 Calcifying odontogenic cyst with ghost cells.

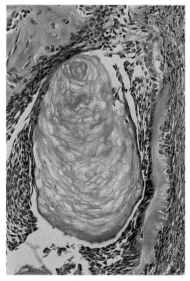

Fig. 72 Calcifying odontogenic cyst with ghost cells.

Cysts without epithelial lining
(non-odontogenic)

Solitary bone cyst

Incidence and aetiology

Rare. Peak age incidence in second decade. Aetiology speculative. Traditionally thought to be traumatic (earlier terms: haemorrhagic or traumatic bone cyst), but no supporting evidence.

Pathology

Almost invariably in mandible. Cavity and radiolucency extends through cancellous bone and arches up between roots of teeth but rarely expands the bone.

May contain serosanguinous fluid or be empty except for air.

Wall usually rough, bare bone sometimes with traces of connective tissue as incomplete lining often with evidence of small haemorrhages. Unlike true cysts, solitary bone cysts probably heal spontaneously. Cavity should be opened only to confirm the diagnosis. The resulting bleeding into the cavity causes it to heal; it is an incorrect assumption that these cysts are *caused* by bleeding into the bone.

Aneurysmal bone cyst

Aetiology

Speculative. Possibly a developmental defect or bleeding into, or vascularisation of, pre-existing lesion such as giant cell granuloma.

Pathology

Grossly, resembles a blood-filled sponge. Microscopically consists of blood-filled spaces lined by flattened cells and separated by highly vascular connective tissue septa and similar solid area often with many giant cells. Sometimes solid areas may calcify and resemble ossifying fibroma.

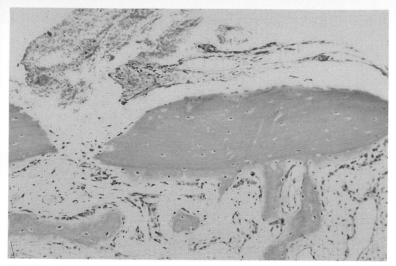

Fig. 73 Solitary bone cyst, scanty incomplete lining (above).

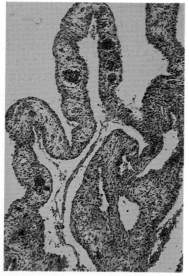

Fig. 74 Aneurysmal bone cyst.

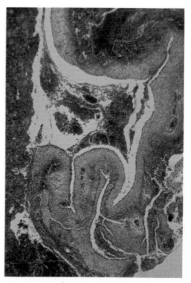

Fig. 75 Aneurysmal bone cyst.

Ameloblastoma

About 80% in ramus or posterior body of mandible. Mainly found in males over 40. Typically produces multiloculated cystic appearance on radiographs but can mimic dental or dentigerous cysts.
Slow growing. (Truly malignant variants are a pathological curiosity.) Locally invasive. Does not metastasise.

Microscopy

Variable appearances, but classically consists of ameloblast-like columnar cells surrounding loosely arranged stellate cells in plexiform (ramifying stands of tumour) or follicular pattern. Microcystic change common either within the epithelial processes or in connective tissue stroma.
Expansion of cysts can overgrow and surround the solid area of tumour leaving no more than mural thickening. Tumour cells forming cyst wall can become so flattened as to resemble lining of simple non-neoplastic cysts.

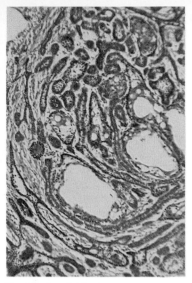

Fig. 76 Ameloblastoma.

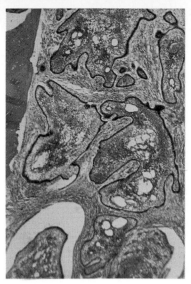

Fig. 77 Ameloblastoma: follicular pattern.

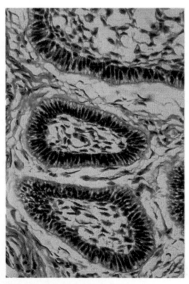

Fig. 78 Ameloblastoma: ameloblast-like cells.

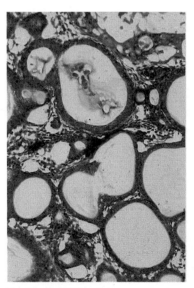

Fig. 79 Ameloblastoma: stromal cysts.

Ameloblastoma (cont)

Degenerative changes producing eosinophilic granular cells may develop.

Squamous metaplasia usually only in small foci but rarely, widespread in the so-called acanthomatous ameloblastoma.

Tumour spreads slowly, mainly through cancellous bone but eventually expands the jaw and can erode through into soft tissue. Often erodes roots of related teeth.

Radical excision is curative, otherwise recurrences develop. Lower border of jaw, however, usually not invaded and may be left intact and mutilating operation avoided.

Close radiographic follow-up needed and any eventual recurrence dealt with as necessary.

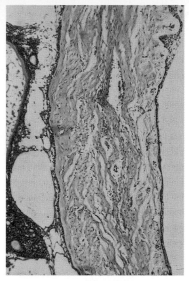

Fig. 80 Cystic ameloblastoma.

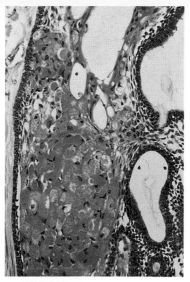

Fig. 81 Ameloblastoma: granular cells.

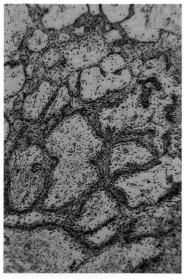

Fig. 82 Acanthomatous ameloblastoma.

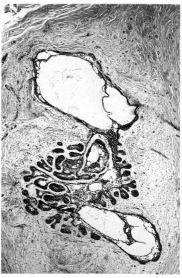

Fig. 83 Soft tissue ameloblastoma.

Adenomatoid odontogenic tumour

Mainly found in the teens or the third decade, and has a higher incidence in women than in men. Usually anterior maxilla.
Surrounds or is contiguous with tooth, producing radiographic appearance similar to dental or dentigerous cyst

Microscopy

Consists of whorls or sheets of small dark epithelial cells frequently with amorphous or crystalline calcifications and microcysts lined by ameloblast-like columnar epithelium.
Fibrous capsule.
Readily enucleated without risk of recurrence.

Calcifying odontogenic 'cyst'

Solid variant of lesion described earlier (p. 35).

Calcifying epithelial odontogenic (Pindborg) tumour (CEOT)

Rare but important because of resemblance to and risk of confusion with poorly differentiated carcinoma. Age and site distribution similar to that of ameloblastoma.
Variable radiographic appearances—circumscribed or diffuse radiolucency often with scattered snow-shower opacities. Variable trabeculation, multilocular, honeycomb or monolocular.

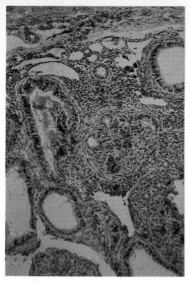

Fig. 84 Adenomatoid odontogenic tumour.

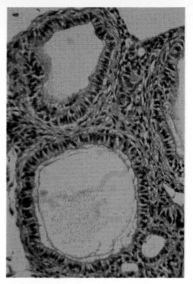

Fig. 85 Adenomatoid odontogenic tumour, microcysts and ameloblast-like cells.

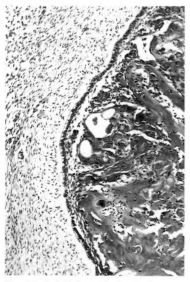

Fig. 86 Calcifying odontogenic 'cyst', solid type.

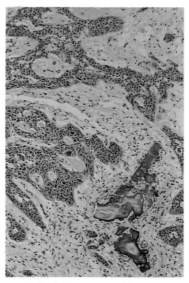

Fig. 87 Calcifying epithelial odontogenic tumour (CEOT).

Calcifying epithelial odontogenic (Pindborg) tumour (CEOT) (cont)

Microscopy

Sheets of variable size squamous cells typically with well-defined cell membranes and prominent intercellular bridges. Nuclei often pleomorphic, large and hyperchromatic resembling carcinoma, or smaller and more uniform. Variations in appearance do not appear to affect behaviour. Clear cells may be present in a few foci or form bulk of tumour. Connective tissue stroma, unlike carcinomas, lacks an inflammatory infiltrate.

Tumour also may contain calcifications and, characteristically, deposits of amyloid. Behaviour probably rather similar to that of ameloblastoma with slow but invasive growth and tendency to recur if not fully excised.

Melanotic neuroectodermal jaw tumour of infancy (progonoma; melano-ameloblastoma)

Rare tumour probably originating from neural crest. Usually detected as ragged area of radiolucency in maxilla at about 3 months; Mandible or other sites rarely affected.

Microscopy

Consists of connective tissue stroma containing foci of pigmented (melanin-containing) cells with pale nuclei surrounding small spaces or clefts together with groups of non-pigmented cells alone or surrounded by pigmented cells.

Variable rate of growth, but most appear to be benign and with rare exceptions do not recur after excision.

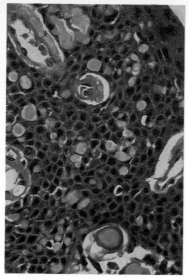

Fig. 88 CEOT with calcifications.

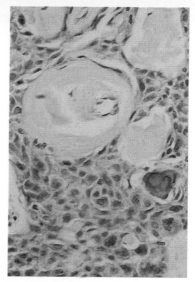

Fig. 89 CEOT amyloid deposits and nuclear pleomorphism.

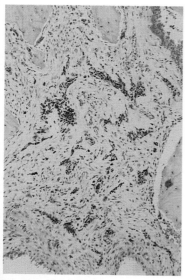

Fig. 90 Progonoma.

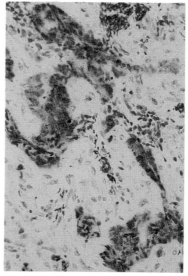

Fig. 91 Progonoma—pigment cells. (High power.)

Ameloblastic fibroma

Exceedingly rare. Typically affects teenagers.
Slow growing, painless swelling and cyst-like
area of radiolucency.

Microscopy

Processes of epithelium resembling ameloblasts
surround cells resembling stellate reticulum.
Stroma resembles dentine papilla.
Thought to be a true mixed tumour.
Sometimes associated with developing
composite odontome.
Readily enucleated but may recur.

Squamous odontogenic tumour

Rare tumour consisting of multiple islands of
well-differentiated squamous cells in connective
tissue stroma.
Wide age distribution and no apparent sex or
site predilection.
Probably minimal risk of recurrence if
conservatively excised.

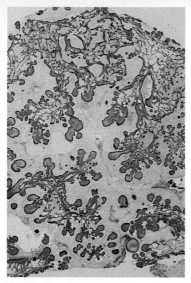

Fig. 92 Ameloblastic fibroma.

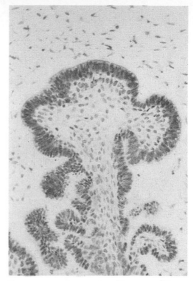

Fig. 93 Ameloblastic fibroma. (High power.)

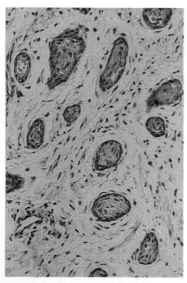

Fig. 94 Squamous odontogenic tumour.

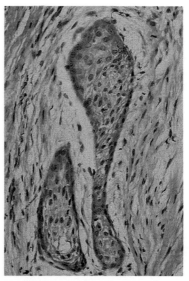

Fig. 95 Squamous odontogenic tumour. (High power.)

Odontogenic myxoma

Probably arises from mesenchymal component of tooth germ.
Usually detected in second or third decade, slightly more frequently in the mandible, as cyst-like or soap-bubble area of radiolucency and expansion of bone.

Microscopy

Loose mucoid fibrillary tissue contains spindle or stellate cells with long delicate intertwining processes and rarely, rests of odontogenic epithelium scattered throughout the tumour. Sometimes extensive bone invasion.
Although benign, this tumour is difficult to remove completely and wide excision is necessary. However, tumour can persist for years or decades afterwards, though without necessarily causing trouble.

Cementomas and cemental dysplasias

Cementoblastoma
Usually males under 25. Radiopaque apical mass usually in molar region with radiolucent margin.

Microscopy

Rounded or irregular mass of cementum on root. Cementum in Pagetoid ('mosaic') pattern with many cementoblasts, peripheral zone of pericementum and zone of uncalcified cement matrix (precementum) and fibrous pericementum.
Probably a benign tumour.

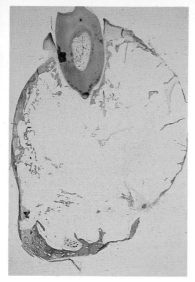

Fig. 96 Odontogenic myxoma.

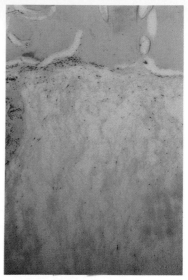

Fig. 97 Odontogenic myxoma—bone invasion.

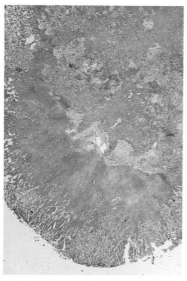

Fig. 98 Cementoblastoma (periphery).

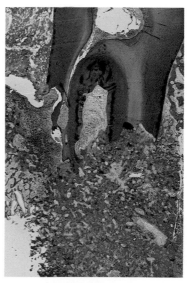

Fig. 99 Cementoblastoma: resorption of related tooth.

Cementomas and cemental dysplasias (cont)

Cementifying fibroma
Most often found in the middle-aged and in molar region. Rounded area of radiolucency resembling apical granuloma but tooth vital. Eventually becomes a radiopaque mass. Enlarging nodules of cementum (cementicles) in fibrous mass which finally becomes densely calcified and progress ceases.

Periapical cemental dysplasia
Somewhat similar to cementifying fibroma but typically in incisor region in middle-aged women.

Gigantiform cementoma
Mainly affects middle-aged black women. Multiple rounded masses resembling secondary cementum near apices particularly of molars and often symmetrical. May expand jaw.

Odontomes (odontomas)

Most are malformations of developing dental tissues (hamartomas). Occasionally associated with a tumour such as ameloblastic fibroma.

Composite odontomes
Compound type. Multiple small tooth-like structures (denticles) within fibrous follicle.
Complex type. Completely irregular mass of dental tissues. May have cauliflower form with dental tissues surrounding a much branched pulp chamber. Though lacking any morphological resemblance to a tooth, complex odontomes have the individual dental tissues in normal relation to one another. Growth ceases when calcification is complete and the mass tends to erupt and frequently then becomes infected.

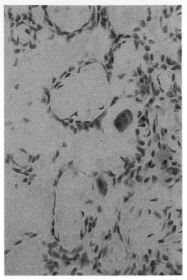

Fig. 100 Cementoblastoma: cementoblasts and giant cells.

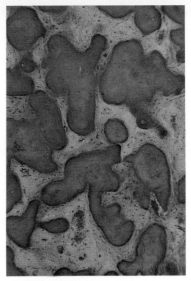

Fig. 101 Cementifying fibroma.

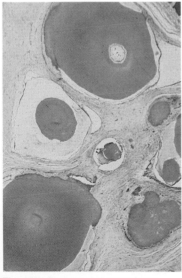

Fig. 102 Compound composite odontome.

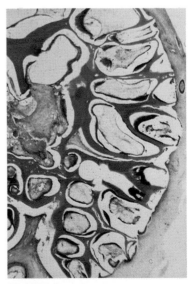

Fig. 103 Complex composite odontome.

Ossifying fibroma

Typically in mid 30s; women twice as frequently affected as men; mandible usually affected. Cellular fibrous tissue containing specks or globules of calcification progressively increasing in size and fusing to form bony masses. Produces circumscribed rounded area of radiolucency with irregular calcifications but increasingly widespread radiopacity.

Chondroma

One of the rarest jaw tumours. Consists of hyaline cartilage containing small chondrocytes in characteristic lacunae. Difficult to distinguish from low grade chondrosarcoma.

Osteoma

May be endosteal or more often periosteal but then often difficult to distinguish from exostoses.
1. *Compact osteoma*. Lamellae of dense compact bone with relatively few osteocytes.
2. *Cancellous*. Widely spaced bony trabeculae with cortex of lamellated bone.

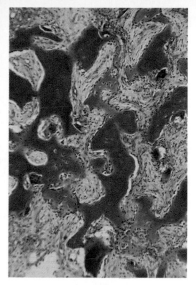

Fig. 104 Ossifying fibroma.

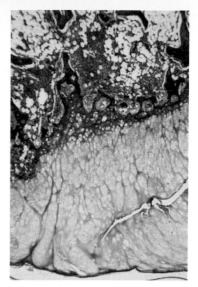

Fig. 105 Osteochondroma.

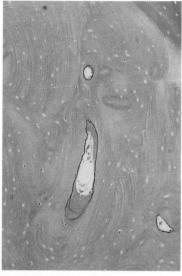

Fig. 106 Compact osteoma.

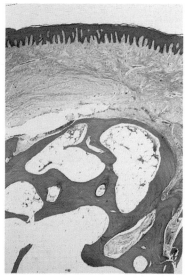

Fig. 107 Cancellous osteoma.

Osteosarcoma

The most common *primary* tumour of bone. Rare complication of radiotherapy or Paget's disease of axial skeleton.
Usually affects young persons, particularly males.

Microscopy

Variable characteristics, and either predominantly osteolytic (undifferentiated) or productive, and then may be predominantly osteochondroblastic or fibroblastic.
Consists of abnormal tumour osteoblasts, typically angular hyperchromatic and larger than normal; often in large numbers in some areas.
Tumour osteoid and bone often formed and predominant in osteoblastic type.
Amounts may be small in chondro- or fibroblastic variants. Sometimes highly vascular or 'telangiectatic'. Destruction of surrounding normal bone.
Histological characteristics do not seem to correlate well with prognosis.
Highly variable radiographic features corresponding with variable histopathology but typically a rapidly growing and painful lesion showing ragged area of radiolucency and radiopacity without definable pattern.
Current treatment wide excision and chemotherapy; not radiosensitive.
5-year survival rate of mandibular tumours about 40%.

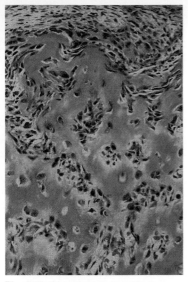

Fig. 108 Osteosarcoma with tumour osteoid.

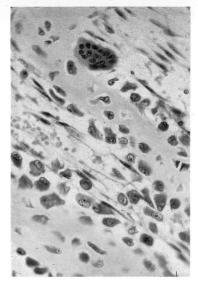

Fig. 109 Osteosarcoma: malignant osteoclasts.

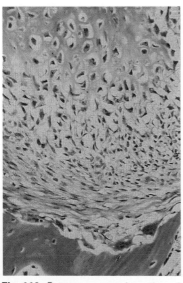

Fig. 110 Osteosarcoma: invasion of normal bone.

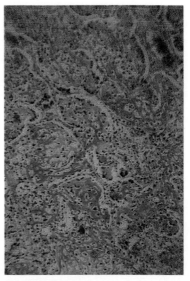

Fig. 111 Osteosarcoma: secondary in lung.

Central giant cell granuloma of the jaws

Aetiology

Unknown. *Not* a neoplasm. Mistakenly termed 'reparative giant cell granuloma' in the past (but more destructive than reparative). No evidence of traumatic aetiology. No changes in blood chemistry. Adolescents or young adults mainly affected, especially females—usually the mandible. Produces area of radiolucency often with faint trabeculation and indefinite borders or soap bubble appearance.

Microscopy

Loose, usually highly cellular and vascular connective tissue stroma containing multinucleate giant cells of variable size. Not histologically distinguishable from bone lesions of hyperparathyroidism. Occasionally rapid growth and corresponding extension of bone destruction, but benign and responds to conservative resection. Residual areas may resolve spontaneously.

Myeloma (plasmacytoma), solitary and multiple

Myeloma is a malignant tumour of plasma cells. These are progeny of B lymphocytes, but myeloma (unlike lymphoma) is usually a destructive bone tumour. Solitary plasmacytomas are rare and may be in soft tissue. Most ultimately become multiple.

Microscopy

The tumour consists of neoplastic plasma cells which produce monoclonal immunoglobulin— usually IgG. Amyloid formation both within the tumour and in other sites, such as the tongue, may result. Myeloma is usually recognised as a result of painful, punched-out bone lesions or pathological fractures.
Occasionally detected early, by chance finding of monoclonal hypergammaglobulinaemia during routine haematological investigation.

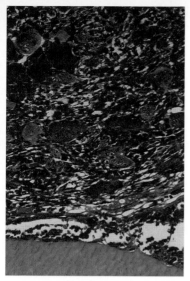

Fig. 112 Central giant cell granuloma.

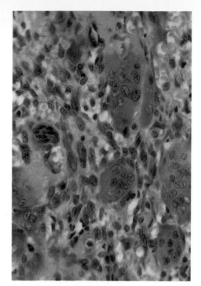

Fig. 113 Giant cell granuloma: typical 'osteoblasts'.

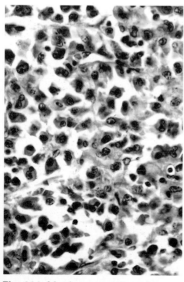

Fig. 114 Myeloma: tumour plasma cells.

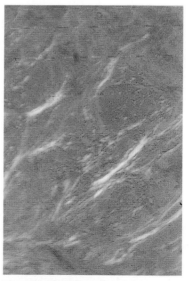

Fig. 115 Myeloma: amyloid deposits in soft tissues.

Eosinophilic granuloma
(histiocytosis X)

A rare tumour-like lesion of bone often first detected in the jaw. It arises from Langerhans cells (the epithelial counterparts of histiocytes) and produces areas of bone destruction. Occasionally tissue destruction is at first mainly of periodontal tissues, exposing the roots of teeth. Eosinophilic granuloma may be solitary or multiple.

Microscopy

The mass consists of pleomorphic histiocytes and eosinophils in dense clusters or thinly scattered. Histiocytes are typically large and pale and variable in size and shape.
Solitary eosinophilic granuloma of the jaw often responds well to wide excision followed by chemotherapy, but the prognosis is somewhat unpredictable.

Hand-Schuller-Christian disease
This is a triad of osteolytic lesions of the skull, exophthalmos and diabetes insipidus due to multifocal eosinophilic granuloma and is a rare variant.

Letterer-Siwe disease
This was thought to be a more malignant form of histiocytosis X affecting infants. Many now believe it to be some other form of lymphoreticular tumour.

Secondary tumours

Carcinomatous metastases are overall the most common tumours of bone but considerably less common in the jaws. Secondaries can come particularly from carcinomas of the breast, lung, prostate, thyroid or kidney and are recognisable by their resemblance to the primary tumour. A deposit in the jaw is very rarely the first sign of a distant asymptomatic primary.

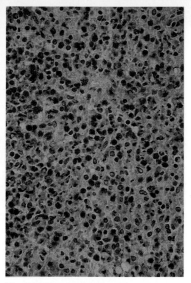

Fig. 116 Eosinophilic granuloma.

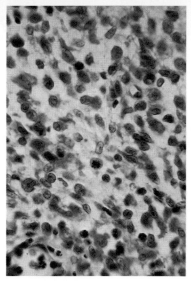

Fig. 117 Eosinophilic granuloma. (High power.)

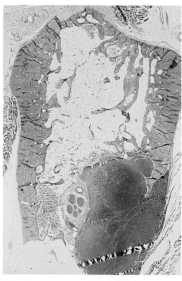

Fig. 118 Secondary carcinoma in mandible.

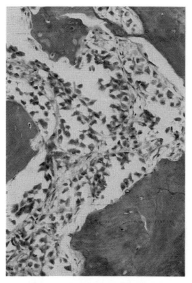

Fig. 119 Secondary deposit of bronchial carcinoma in jaw.

Non-neoplastic Bone Diseases (1)

Fibrous dysplasia (monostotic)

Unknown aetiology. Maxilla frequently affected. Painless rounded swelling; ill-defined margins. Ground glass radiolucency but increasing radiopacity with ill-defined margins.

Microscopy

Rounded focus of fibrous tissue in place of normal bone. Alternating formation and resorption of fine trabeculae of woven bone in 'Chinese letter' pattern with small scattered foci of giant cells.

Progressively increasing ossification and, typically, arrest of progress with maturation of skeleton.

No significant changes in blood chemistry.

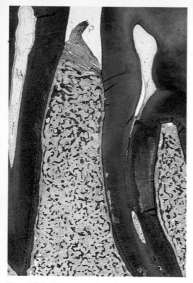

Fig. 120 Fibrous dysplasia involving periodontal tissues.

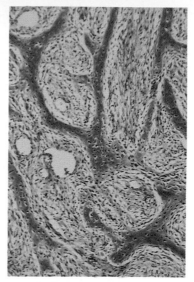

Fig. 121 Fibrous dysplasia: trabeculae of woven bone.

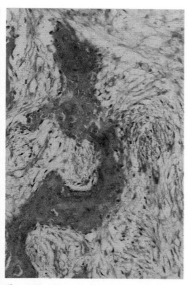

Fig. 122 Fibrous dysplasia: detail of woven bone.

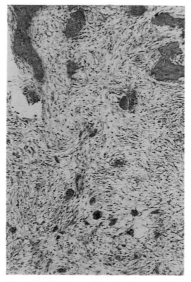

Fig. 123 Fibrous dysplasia: small focus of giant cells.

Non-neoplastic Bone Diseases (2)

Cherubism (familial fibrous dysplasia)

Resembles fibrous dysplasia in cessation of progress after skeletal maturation but differs in (a) microscopic features (b) symmetrical involvement of jaws (mandible, ramus and adjacent body; maxilla also in severe cases) (c) lesions appear multicystic on radiographs (d) dominant inheritance in some cases.

Microscopy

Replacement of bone by loose vascular connective tissue containing many giant cells usually resembling giant cell granuloma. Histopathology of cherubism and fibrous dysplasias is not in itself diagnostic. Confirmation depends on
1. Clinical picture
2. Radiographic features
3. Behaviour of lesion.

Hyperparathyroidism

Aetiology

Primary hyperparathyroidism—hypersecretion of parathormone by parathyroid tumour but bone lesions now exceedingly rare. Secondary hyperparathyroidism results from renal failure leading to reactive parathyroid hyperplasia.

Microscopy

Tumour-like foci of osteoclasts produce cyst-like areas (sometimes multilocular) on radiographs (osteitis fibrosa cystica). Microscopically indistinguishable from giant cell granuloma of the jaws. Diagnosis depends on serum chemistry changes, namely, raised calcium (up to $\times 2$ normal), normal or low phosphate and raised alkaline phosphatase.

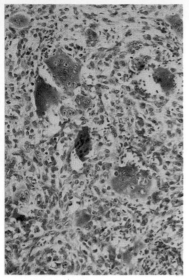

Fig. 124 Cherubism.

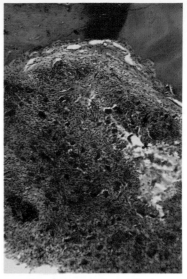

Fig. 125 Hyperparathyroidism.

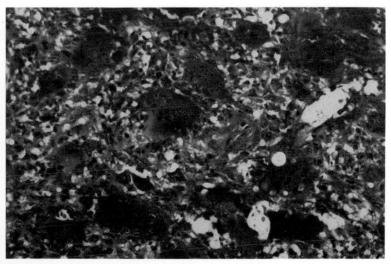

Fig. 126 Hyperparathyroidism: details of osteoclasts.

Non-neoplastic Bone Diseases (3)

Paget's disease of bone (osteitis deformans)

Aetiology and prevalence

May affect, in some degree, 5% of population over 55 in Britain. Aetiology unknown but some evidence for a viral cause.
Pelvis, calvarium and limbs mainly affected. Maxilla occasionally and mandible rarely affected. Lesions predominantly osteolytic initially, but increasing sclerosis, often with gross generalised thickening of bone with cotton wool appearance.
Greatly raised serum alkaline phosphatase (up to 100 KAu/ml).

Microscopy

Anarchic disorganisation of normal bone remodelling with alternating resorption and deposition: many osteoblasts and osteoclasts line bone margins. Irregular pattern of reversal lines produces jigsaw-puzzle ('mosaic') pattern of basophilic lines in the bone.
Increased risk of sarcomatous change later, but hardly ever in the jaws.

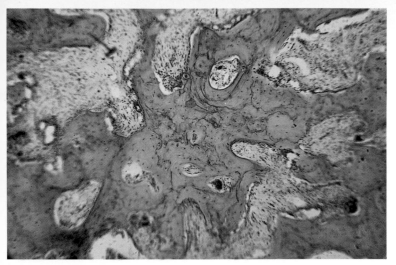

Fig. 127 Paget's disease of bone.

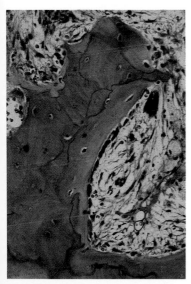

Fig. 128 Paget's disease of bone: 'mosaic' (reversal) lines.

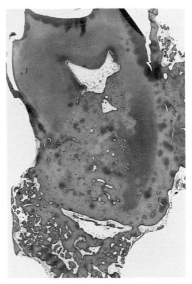

Fig. 129 Paget's disease: irregular hypercementosis of tooth.

Non-neoplastic Bone Diseases (4)

Radiation injury (osteoradionecrosis)

Irradiation for cancer of this region can cause death of bone cells leaving empty lacunae and obliterative endarteritis, leaving severely ischaemic areas of bone. Attempts to separate this dead tissue by osteoclasts produce moth-eaten areas but this activity is limited by the poor blood supply. Infection, usually from teeth, readily spreads in the ischaemic bone and can give rise to extensive chronic osteomyelitis.

Osteomyelitis

Aetiology

Infection of the jaw can rarely result from severe dental infections or from fractures open to the skin or secondary to irradiation.

Microscopy

Infection spreads through the cancellous spaces leading to thrombosis of blood vessels in bony canaliculae and bone necrosis.
Necrotic bone shows empty lacunae, is typically infiltrated by inflammatory cells and may show masses of bacteria. Osteoblasts from healthy peripheral bone resorb the junction with infected bone which becomes separated as a sequestrum.

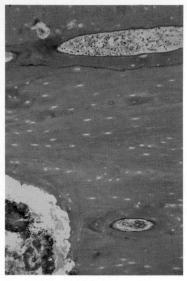

Fig. 130 Osteoradionecrosis.

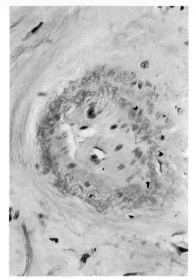

Fig. 131 Irradiation-induced obliterative endarteritis in bone.

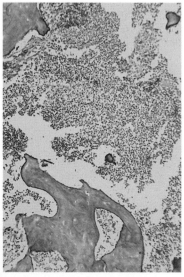

Fig. 132 Acute osteomyelitis. Dead bone and inflammatory cells.

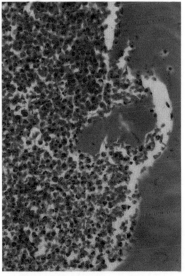

Fig. 133 Acute osteomyelitis: acute inflammatory cells in dead bone.

| # Infective Stomatitis

Herpetic stomatitis

Aetiology

A primary infection of a non-immune individual by HSV (usually) type 1. Steadily declining incidence in developed countries. Increased prevalence in immunodeficiency, e.g. AIDS.

Pathology

Viral infection of epithelial cells produces intra-epithelial vesicles with viral-damaged cells in the floor leading to epithelial destruction, ulcers and inflammation.
Smears from early lesions show ballooning degeneration of epithelial cell nuclei (viral proliferation pushing chromatin to form peripheral rim) and epithelial giant cells.
Systemic febrile illness, lymphadenopathy, and rising titre of antibodies.

Herpes labialis
Virus may persist in trigeminal ganglion. Periodic reactivation leads to vesicles and crusting ulcers on borders of lips in about 30% after primary infection. Microscopic features the same as for primary infection.

Herpes zoster of the trigeminal area

Reactivation infection by varicella-zoster virus usually long after the initial infection (chickenpox). Skin and mucosa of the trigeminal sensory area affected. Lesions clinically and histologically the same as those of herpes simplex.

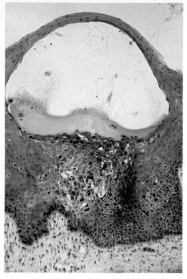

Fig. 134 Herpetic stomatitis: intact vesicle.

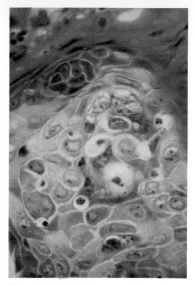

Fig. 135 Herpetic stomatitis: virus-damaged cells in floor of vesicle.

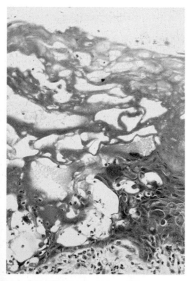

Fig. 136 Herpetic stomatitis: necrosis of epithelium.

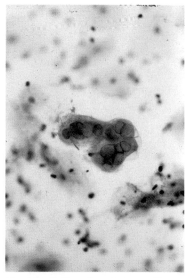

Fig. 137 Ballooning degeneration of epithelial cells in smear.

Non-specific ulceration can result from trauma or unidentified causes as in recurrent aphthae.

Recurrent aphthae

Aetiology

Unknown aetiology in most cases. Many reported immunological abnormalities but aetiological significance doubtful. Not an autoimmune disease—affects otherwise healthy persons, and not associated with recognised autoimmune diseases. No useful immunological diagnostic tests. No reliable response to immunosuppressive treatment. In 5–10%, ulcers precipitated by deficiency of, and respond to administration of, folate, vitamin B_{12} or occasionally iron. 10–20% of the population are affected in some degree.
Typically starts mildly in childhood or adolescence and often peaks in early adult life and then gradually declines. Rare onset late in life usually associated with deficiency state.

Microscopy

Ulceration appears to be preceded by leucocytic infiltration of the epithelium and underlying corium and intercellular oedema leading to disintegration of the epithelium. Ulcers have no specific features but consist of a break in the epithelium with an intense inflammatory infiltrate extending deeply. Diagnosis therefore depends largely on the history of regular recurrences and clinical features.

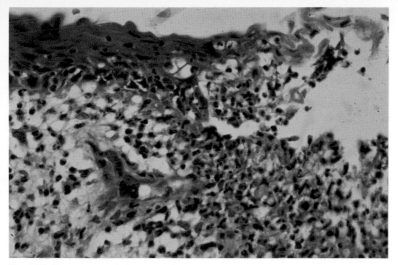

Fig. 138 Recurrent aphtha: margin.

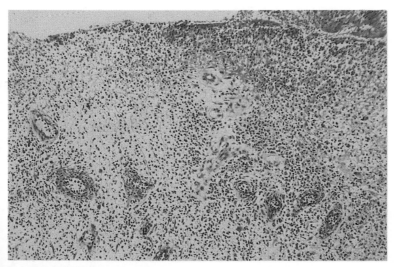

Fig. 139 Aphtha: centre of ulcer.

Lichen planus

Aetiology

Unknown. Possibly immunologically mediated but typically in otherwise healthy persons and not associated with other such diseases. In a minority results from drug treatment (gold, antimalarials, methyldopa, etc.). Most common after 45. About 65% of cases in females. Cutaneous lichen planus often minimal or not associated.

Microscopy

Oral lesions are of 3 types, often all associated.
1. *Striae (white lesions)*. Hyper- or parakeratosis is associated with pointed, sometimes saw-tooth rete ridges, liquefaction degeneration of the basal cell layer and a band-like mononuclear (predominantly T lymphocyte) infiltrate with a well-defined lower border in the corium. These 'classical' changes are not often all found together.
2. *Atrophic (red) lesions*. The epithelium is thin and flattened without keratosis. The inflammatory infiltrate is more dense but still band-like.
3. *Erosions*. The epithelium is destroyed by progression of atrophy (**not** by rupture of bullae). Secondary infection increases the inflammatory response and produces a non-specific picture apart from any changes of lichen planus at the margins.

Prognosis

Lichen planus, though usually a self-limiting disease, can persist for many years if untreated. Responds well to potent corticosteroids. The risk of malignant change remains controversial.

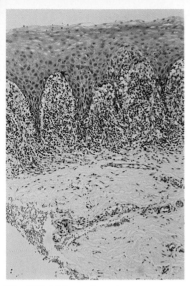

Fig. 140 Lichen planus.

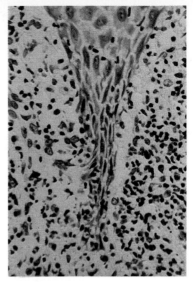

Fig. 141 Lichen planus: detail of liquefaction degeneration of basal cells.

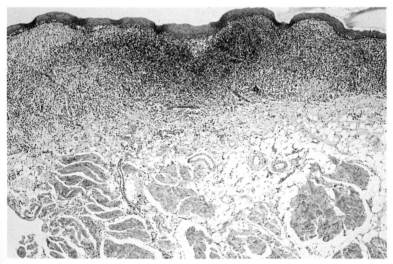

Fig. 142 Lichen planus: atrophic type.

Bullous erythema multiforme
(Stevens-Johnson syndrome)

Aetiology

Unknown, but occasionally follows drug treatment (especially long-acting sulphonamides) or herpetic infection. Most cases are 'idiopathic'. No immunological mechanism identified. Typically affects young adults and tends to recur two or three times a year then spontaneously resolves after a time. Rarely severe multisystem illness with fatal renal involvement.

Mucocutaneous vesiculobullous disease but often only oral involvement of significant degree. Skin—bullae or target lesions; eyes—conjunctivitis or iritis; mouth—swollen, crusted, bleeding lips and widespread ill-defined oral erosions.

Microscopy

Variable picture with degeneration of spinous cells and widespread intercellular oedema, sometimes leading to intra-epithelial vesiculation or extensive vacuolar change leading to subepithelial vesiculation.

Rupture of vesicles leaves erosions. There is a mononuclear inflammatory infiltrate subepithelially and around superficial blood vessels.

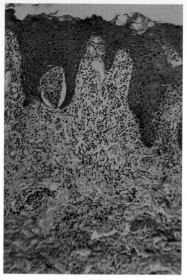

Fig. 143 Bullous erythema multiforme, early stage.

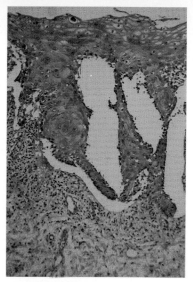

Fig. 144 Erythema multiforme: progressive separation of epithelium.

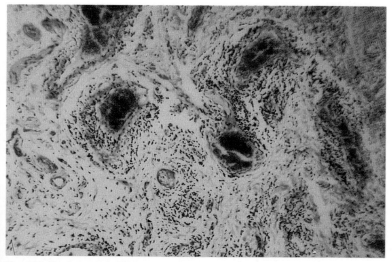

Fig. 145 Erythema multiforme: perivascular inflammatory infiltrate.

Pemphigus vulgaris

Aetiology and pathology

A 'typical' autoimmune disease with circulating autoantibodies against epithelial intercellular cement substance, which can also be localised by immunofluorescence. Destruction of intercellular adherence leads to disintegration of epithelia and intra-epithelial vesiculation, often first in the mouth. Widespread skin lesions are fatal from loss of fluid and electrolytes and infection, but controllable with heavy immunosuppressive treatment. Women are more frequently affected, usually between the ages of 40 and 50.

Microscopy

Separation of epithelial cells from one another (acantholysis) initially forming suprabasal clefts then intra-epithelial vesicles with rounded acantholytic cells floating in the vesicle fluid. Rupture of vesicles leaves ulcers.
There is positive immunofluorescence of immunoglobulin (usually IgG) along intercellular junctions and coating detached acantholytic cells.

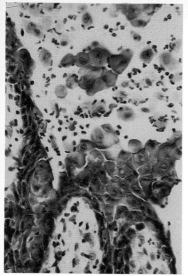

Fig. 146 Pemphigus vulgaris: acantholytic cells separating—early stage.

Fig. 147 Pemphigus vulgaris: immunoflorescence showing IgG along intercellular borders of epithelium.

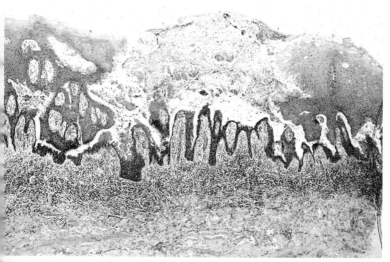

Fig. 148 Pemphigus vulgaris: recently ruptured vesicle.

Mucous membrane pemphigoid

Aetiology and pathology

Some evidence for immunopathogenesis with formation of autoantibodies against basement membrane, but not frequently detectable in serum and only detectable in target area in about 40%. Complement (C3) is detectable subepithelially however in about 80%.
No recognised association with other autoimmune diseases.
Women usually over middle-age predominantly affected.

Microscopy

Subepithelial bulla formation leads to detachment of areas of full thickness of epithelium from the corium, which becomes infiltrated with inflammatory cells.
Immunoglobulin or complement may be detectable along basement membrane by immunofluorescence.
The main sequel is scar formation after healing of erosions. In the eyes this can damage sight.

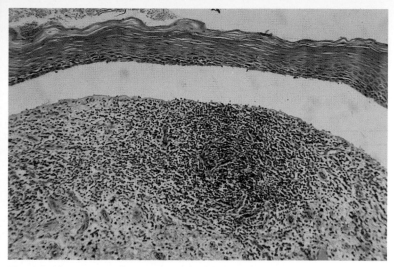

Fig. 149 Mucous membrane pemphigoid.

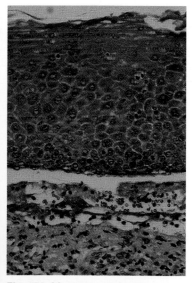

Fig. 150 Mucous membrane pemphigoid. (High power.)

Fig. 151 Mucous membrane pemphigoid: immunofluorescence of complement (C3) along basement membrane zone.

Lupus erythematosus

Aetiology and pathology

Both systemic (SLE) and discoid (DLE) types can produce oral lesions somewhat resembling those of lichen planus clinically.

SLE is characterised by a wide variety of circulating autoantibodies, particularly antinuclear factors and often rheumatoid factor. Thought to be immune-complex mediated, and multisystem involvement with arthritis as the most common feature. DLE is a mucocutaneous disease with epithelial lesions indistinguishable from those of SLE but without significant autoantibody production. Women often between 20 and 30 chiefly affected.

Microscopy

Highly variable picture with wildly irregular patterns of acanthosis or epithelial atrophy, liquefaction degeneration of the basal cell layer and widely scattered inflammatory infiltrate in the corium. Thickening of basement membrane zone shown by PAS staining. Immunoglobulin and complement also detectable there by immunofluorescence.

ORAL PATHOLOGY

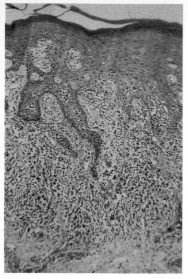

Fig. 152 Lupus erythematosus.

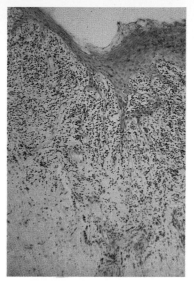

Fig. 153 Lupus erythematosus: adjacent epithelial atrophy and acanthosis.

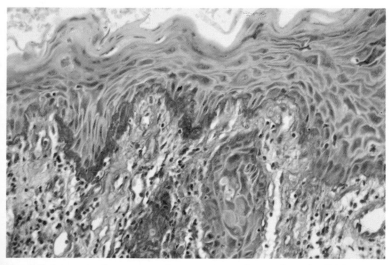

Fig. 154 Lupus erythematosus: basement membrane deposits (PAS stain.)

14 | Keratoses (Leukoplakias; White Lesions) (1)

Terminology

Oral white plaques share many histological features, and idiopathic forms (leukoplakia) are often not distinguishable histologically from those with defined causes such as frictional keratosis but may show dysplasia. More frequently, features of oral white lesions include the following in varying combinations:

Microscopy

1. Hyper(ortho)keratosis—a superficial eosinophilic layer of dead epithelial squames under which there is a layer of epithelial cells containing basophilic granules of prekeratin.
2. Parakeratosis—the surface consists of effete epithelial cells containing shrunken, pyknotic, basophilic nuclei with no underlying granular cell layer.
3. Acanthosis—hyperplasia of the prickle cell layer usually with loss of the normally regular profile of the rete ridges.
4. Epithelial atrophy—thinning usually with loss of the rete ridges of the epithelium.
5. Dysplasia (see below) may be associated with keratosis but there is no consistent relationship.

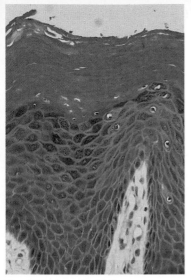

Fig. 155 Hyper(ortho)keratosis.

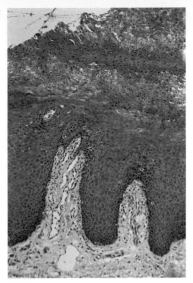

Fig. 156 Parakeratosis and acanthosis.

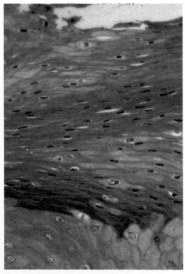

Fig. 157 Parakeratosis: detail.

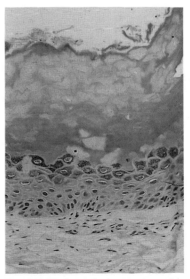

Fig. 158 Hyperorthokeratosis and epithelial atrophy.

14 | Keratoses (Leukoplakias; White Lesions) (2)

White sponge naevus

Aetiology and pathology

Hereditary (autosomal dominant) disorder producing soft white thickening of oral mucosa. Asymptomatic (may not be noticed until adulthood), but tags of protruding epithelium may be chewed off or detached, producing an irregular surface. The whole of the oral mucosa may be affected to variable degree.

Microscopy

Typically regular acanthosis with widespread intracellular oedema extending particularly in the plaque where prominent cell membranes give a 'basket-weave' appearance. The surface is typically irregular. Inflammatory infiltrate is absent from the corium.

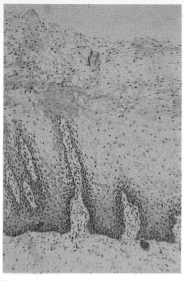

Fig. 159 White sponge naevus.

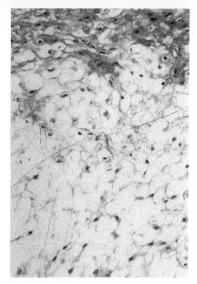

Fig. 160 White sponge naevus: oedematous epithelial cells.

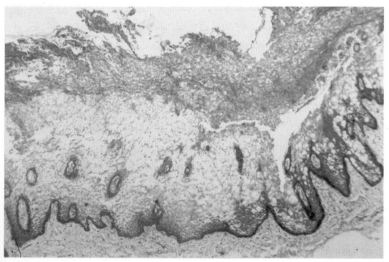

Fig. 161 White sponge naevus: partial detachment of plaque.

Keratoses (Leukoplakias; White Lesions) (3)

Frictional keratosis

This shows non-specific keratosis microscopically and is distinguishable only by clinical evidence of mechanical trauma.

Smoker's keratosis

This results from heavy long-term pipe smoking, is therefore seen mainly in men, and affects the palate. The keratosis is non-specific but there is characteristically inflammation and swelling of the palatal mucous glands producing red umbilicated swellings.

Syphilitic leukoplakia

A feature of the tertiary stage of syphilis but rarely seen now.
Typically affects dorsum of tongue and there is a high risk of malignant change.
Features of epithelial keratosis not specific but dysplasia or malignant change may be evident. Characteristic syphilitic inflammatory response (endarteritis, plasma cell infiltrate and occasionally granuloma formation) may be seen deeply, but diagnosis is essentially serological.

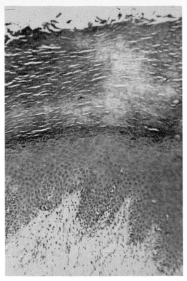

Fig. 162 Frictional keratosis.

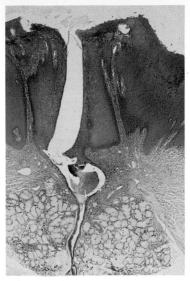

Fig. 163 Smoker's keratosis: swollen palatal salivary tissue.

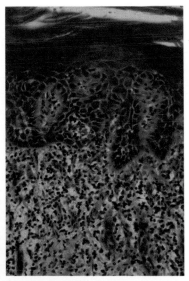

Fig. 164 Syphilitic leukoplakia with mild dysplasia.

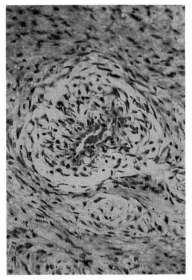

Fig. 165 Endarteritis beneath syphilitic leukoplakia.

Keratoses (Leukoplakias; White Lesions) (4)

Candidosis (thrush)

Aetiology

Acute infection by *Candida albicans*, usually in immunodeficient patients (e.g. neonates, immunosuppressive drugs, AIDS, debilitating illnesses, etc.).

Microscopy

Hyphae invade oral epithelium producing a parakeratotic plaque but with cells separated by inflammatory oedema and neutrophils. Inflammatory infiltrate concentrated at junction of plaque with spinous layer forming micro-abscesses and moderate infiltrate also in the corium. Hyperplasia of rete ridges forms long slender downgrowths.

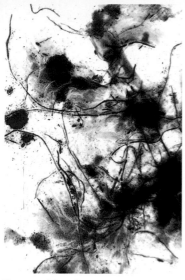

Fig. 166 Thrush: tangled hyphae in smear. (Gram stain.)

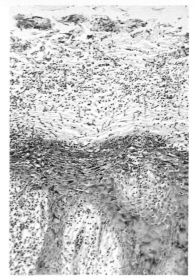

Fig. 167 Thrush: plaque. (PAS.)

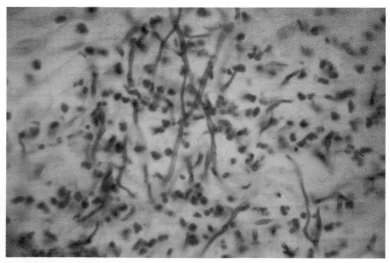

Fig. 168 Thrush: hyphae in plaque. (High power; PAS.)

Keratoses (Leukoplakias; White Lesions) **(5)**

Chronic candidosis (candida leukoplakia)

Uncommon, persistent candidal infection usually of middle-age or over.

Microscopy

Production of parakeratotic plaque. Hyphae grow through plaque to spinous layer. Plaque infiltrated by moderate numbers of leukocytes and beads of oedema. Deeper epithelium acanthotic, sometimes grossly, and sometimes dysplastic.

Chronic mucocutaneous candidosis syndromes

All rare but comprise leukoplakia-like oral candidosis associated with variable skin and nail involvement, and sometimes systemic disorders. Limited defect of cellular immunity in about 60% of patients but no special susceptibility to systemic candidosis.
One variant associated with endocrine deficiencies, particularly primary hypoparathyroidism and Addison's disease (candida endocrinopathy syndrome).

Microscopy

As for isolated chronic candidosis (see Figs. 169–171).

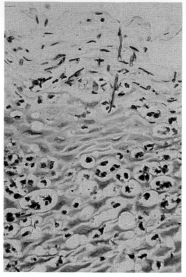

Fig. 169 Chronic candidosis: hyphae invading parakeratotic plaque. (PAS.)

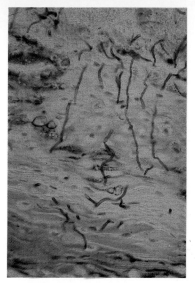

Fig. 170 Chronic candidosis: hyphae and inflammatory infiltrate in plaque.

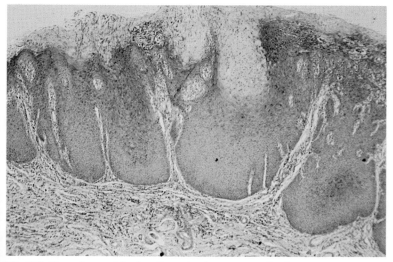

Fig. 171 Chronic candidosis: plaque and gross acanthosis.

Keratoses (Leukoplakias; White Lesions)(6)

Dysplasia (epithelial atypia; dyskeratosis)

Dysplasia is abnormal maturation and differentiation of the epithelium, as seen in carcinomas and also in leukoplakias, when it is usually an indication of premalignancy. The following features are seen in varying combinations:

Microscopy

1. Hyperchromatism and alteration of nuclear cytoplasmic ratio. The nuclei are abnormally large in relation to the area of cytoplasm and are more heavily basophilic. Nucleoli may be more prominent or numerous. Nuclear pleomorphism (irregularly shaped nuclei) is often associated.
2. Individual, deep cell keratinisation (dyskeratosis). Individual cells within the prickle cell layer develop cytoplasmic keratin and become eosinophilic.
3. Loss of polarity. The basal cell layer loses its normal orderly arrangement and the cells lie irregularly at angles to one another.
4. Mitoses. These may be seen superficially among the spinous cells and are of sinister import, particularly if abnormal.
5. Other features. Loss of intercellular adherence with fluid-filled spaces appearing between the epithelial cells and drop-shaped (bulbous) rete ridges are sometimes associated with dysplasia. Hyperkeratosis and/or acanthosis may or may not be associated.

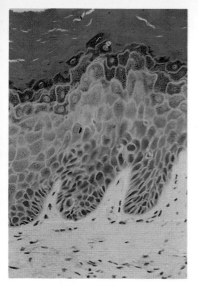

Fig. 172 Mild to moderate dysplasia with hyperchromatism and hyperkeratosis.

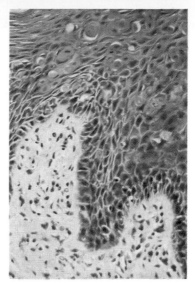

Fig. 173 Dysplasia with deep cell keratinisation: hyperchromatism and loss of polarity.

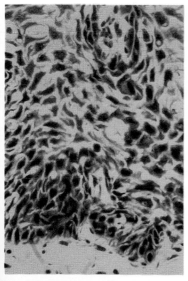

Fig. 174 Dysplasia: loss of intercellular adherence.

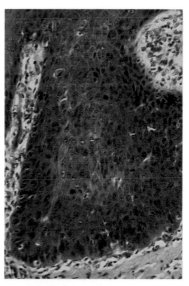

Fig. 175 Severe dysplasia (top to bottom change, carcinoma in situ).

Erythroplasia ('erythroplakia')

This is a clinical term for chronic red lesions (i.e. hyperkeratosis is absent), which are typically level with or depressed below the surrounding mucosa and typically show severe dysplasia or early carcinoma.

Early carcinoma

In addition to dysplastic leukoplakias, some early carcinomas, before ulcerating, produce keratin on the surface and appear as innocent white lesions. Microscopically there is invasive squamous cell carcinoma replacing the normal epithelial surface and an overlying parakeratinised plaque.

Squamous cell papilloma

A common benign lesion characterised by fine finger-like papillae, giving it a characteristic warty appearance clinically.

Microscopy

A central branching core of vascular connective tissue extends into the papillae. The latter are covered by hyperplastic stratified squamous epithelium which may be keratinised. The papilloma then appears white.
Excision is curative.

Adenoma

See Salivary gland tumours (p. 121).

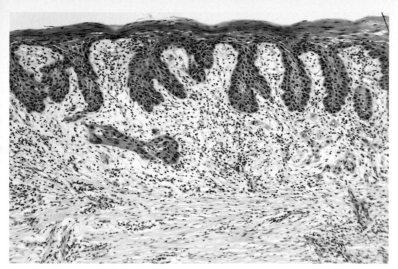

Fig. 176 Erythroplasia.

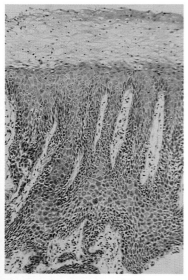

Fig. 177 Carcinoma with keratinised surface.

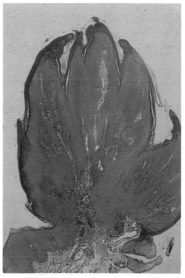

Fig. 178 Squamous cell papilloma.

15 | Squamous Cell Carcinoma (1)

Aetiology and pathology

Aetiological factors usually unidentifiable. In Britain, at least, no association with cigarette-smoking or alcohol consumption—steady increase in their consumption associated with steady *decline* in oral cancer. Possible association with pipe-smoking and high incidence of oral carcinoma in India may be associated with different types and forms of tobacco usage. Usually found after age 50 and incidence increases with age.

Lip cancer associated with excess exposure to sunshine, especially in fair skinned males. Associated with leukoplakia in only a minority.

Microscopy

Essential features are epithelial abnormalities (dysplasia) and invasion. Later, metastases develop, particularly in regional lymph nodes. Most are well differentiated with obvious squamous pattern and formation of whorls of keratin deeply (cell nests).

The basement membrane tends to disappear and the tumour appears as invading, irregular epithelial processes or sheets of cells with ill-defined outlines typically surrounded by chronic inflammatory cells. Invasion is characterised by destruction of tissues in the path of the tumour. Neoplastic epithelial cells are pleomorphic, show variably enlarged, often hyperchromatic nuclei or vesicular nuclei with prominent or multiple nucleoli. Mitoses may be numerous and atypical. With increasing dedifferentiation the neoplastic cells may become progressively more uniformly hyperchromatic and regular in size so that they may become difficult to recognise as carcinomas by light microscopy in extreme (anaplastic) examples.

ORAL PATHOLOGY

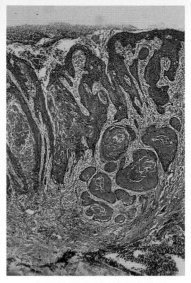

Fig. 179 Squamous cell carcinoma: well-differentiated.

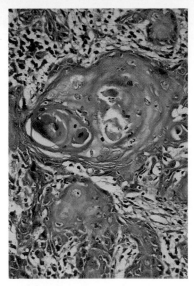

Fig. 180 Squamous carcinoma: cell nest formation.

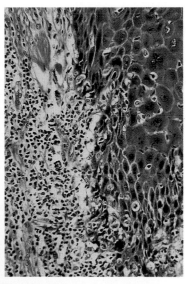

Fig. 181 Squamous carcinoma: dysplasia.

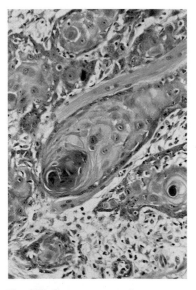

Fig. 182 Squamous carcinoma destroying muscle.

15 | Squamous Cell Carcinoma (2)

Prognosis

The main forms of treatment are wide excision often with radiotherapy, or radiotherapy alone. Good survival rates depend on early diagnosis and treatment. Survival also deteriorates with age. Average 5-year survival rates for carcinoma of the tongue are 37% for males and 46% for females. Most other sites within the mouth have a rather better prognosis.

Carcinoma of the lip has a much better prognosis and a 5-year survival rate of 94% for males but (inexplicably) only 84% for females.

Verrucous carcinoma

An uncommon variant which appears as a prominent white warty plaque.

Microscopy

There is gross hyperkeratosis and papillary epithelial hyperplasia producing a folded appearance with intervening cleft-like spaces. The uniform level of downgrowth of the tumour gives a well-defined deep margin. Epithelial atypia is minimal (in the early stages), but there is typically a chronic inflammatory infiltrate in the corium.

Prognosis

Spread and metastasis is slower than squamous cell carcinoma and response to adequate excision is better. Irradiation however may induce anaplastic change and accelerate growth.

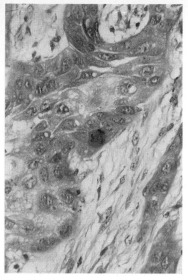

Fig. 183 Squamous carcinoma: abnormal mitoses.

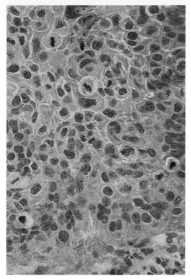

Fig. 184 Poorly-differentiated squamous carcinoma.

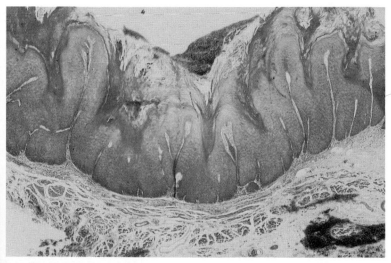

Fig. 185 Verrucous carcinoma.

Fibrous nodules (fibrous epulides, polyps and denture granulomas)

Aetiology and pathology

These are some of the most common oral swellings but are hyperplastic in nature, resulting from fibrous proliferation in response to chronic irritation often with an inflammatory component.

Microscopy

These lesions are distinguishable only by their site of origin and consist of irregular bundles of collagenous connective tissue with varying numbers of fibroblasts covered by stratified squamous epithelium, often with mild subepithelial inflammatory infiltrate. More severe and deeply extending inflammation results from ulceration.
Adequate excision should be curative.

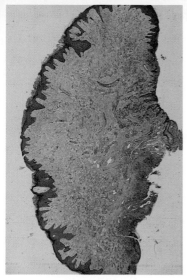

Fig. 186 Fibrous epulis.

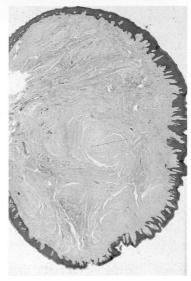

Fig. 187 Fibrous polyp of cheek.

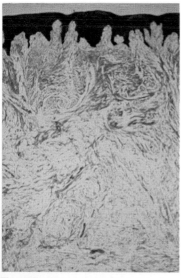

Fig. 188 Fibrous nodule: general structure.

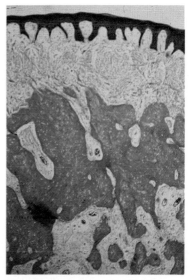

Fig. 189 Bone formation in fibrous epulis.

Pyogenic granuloma

These nodules, which can also affect the skin, consist of loose vascular connective tissue with an intense and acute inflammatory infiltrate and covered with epithelium. An inflamed pregnancy epulis is histologically indistinguishable frcm a pyogenic granuloma.

Pregnancy epulis

Most resemble pyogenic granulomas, but others lack inflammation and consist of dilated thin-walled vessels in an oedematous connective tissue stroma. Presumably this vascular proliferation results from hormonal factors.

Giant cell epulis

A hyperplastic lesion believed to result from proliferation of osteoclasts from the sites of shedding of deciduous teeth as it is only found in this area of the alveolar ridge and mainly in young people.

Microscopy

A mass of osteoclast-like giant cells in a vascular stroma of ovoid or spindle-shaped cells with fine connective tissue fibres and covered by stratified squamous epithelium.

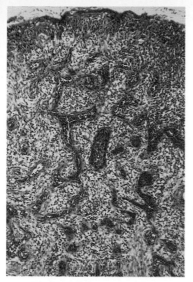

Fig. 190 Pyogenic granuloma.

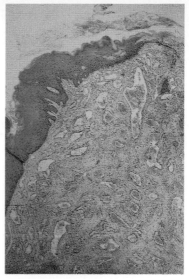

Fig. 191 Pregnancy epulis.

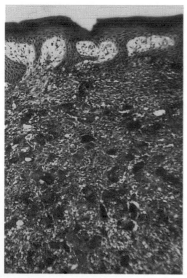

Fig. 192 Giant cell epulis.

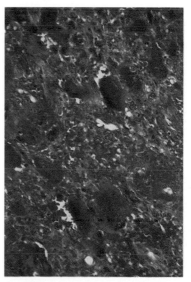

Fig. 193 Giant cell epulis. (High power.)

17 Benign Connective Tissue Tumours (1)

Neurofibroma

Neurofibromas are uncommon tumours arising from nerve sheath fibroblasts and consist of wavy bundles of collagen and fibroblasts with elongated nuclei. Variable amounts of mucinous ground substance are present and may produce a myxoid appearance. Tumour may contain nerve fibres or be continuous with the sheath of a nerve.

Neurilemmoma

Neurilemmomas arise from Schwann cells which form the axonal sheath. They characteristically comprise two types of tissue. Antoni A tissue consists of regularly arranged elongated spindle cells with closely aligned (palisaded) nuclei which are darkly basophilic and elongated. Antoni B areas consist of shorter spindle-shaped or oval cells in a mucinous matrix and wavy delicate bundles of collagen fibres.

Traumatic (amputation) neuroma

Proliferation of fibres from the proximal stump of a severed nerve can produce a tumour-like nodule of nerve fascicles surrounded by fibrous tissue.

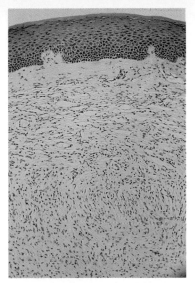

Fig. 194 Neurofibroma.

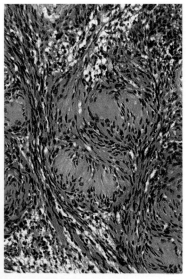

Fig. 195 Neurilemmoma.

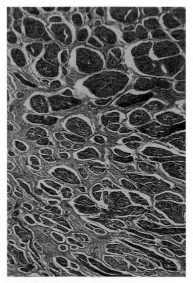

Fig. 196 Traumatic neuroma.

17 | Benign Connective Tissue Tumours (2)

Plexiform neuroma

This consists of a tangled mass of nerve fibres cut in various planes. It can be a solitary lesion or a characteristic feature of neurofibromatosis (von Recklinghausen's disease). When found in the lateral border of the tongue, particularly, this lesion is likely to be one of the features of multiple endocrine adenomatosis and associated with phaeochromocytoma and medullary carcinoma of the thyroid.

Haemangiomas

These are usually hamartomas rather than true tumours and are sometimes part of a widespread developmental defect (mucocutaneous angiomatosis, portwine stain).

Microscopy

Capillary haemangiomas
These consist of a mass of fine capillaries or imperforate rosettes of endothelial cells, covered by squamous epithelium.

Cavernous haemangiomas
These consist of dilated, thin-walled, blood-filled vessels or sinusoids covered by squamous epithelium. If a haemangioma needs to be removed, cryotherapy is probably then the treatment of choice because of the risk of serious haemorrhage.

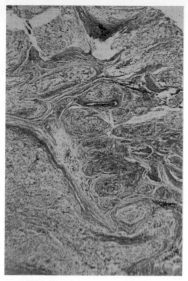

Fig. 197 Plexiform neuroma.

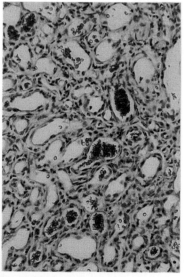

Fig. 198 Capillary haemangioma.

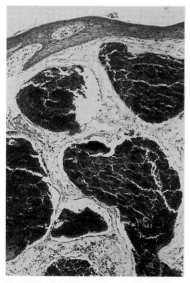

Fig. 199 Cavernous haemangioma.

Benign Connective Tissue Tumours (3)

Lymphangiomas

Generally resemble cavernous haemangiomas but consist of dilated lymphatic vessels which do not contain blood cells unless traumatised.

Vascular leiomyomas

Microscopy

Rare, benign tumours of smooth muscle of vessel walls and consist predominantly of smooth muscle cells which are concentrically arranged around small vessels but spread out without any regular pattern into the main tumour areas.

Lipoma

Lipomas are benign tumours of fat cells and most commonly arise from the buccal fat pad.

Microscopy

The mass consists of fat cells (adipocytes) held together by loose areolar tissue and covered by mucosa.
Excision is curative.
Liposarcomas are recognised but exceedingly rare oral tumours.

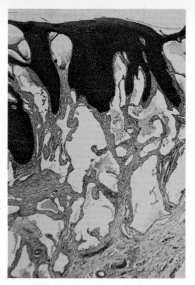

Fig. 200 Lymphangioma.

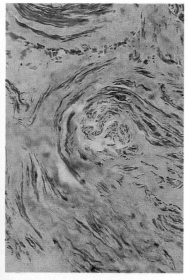

Fig. 201 Vascular leiomyoma. (PTAH stain.)

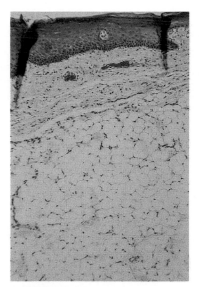

Fig. 202 Lipoma.

Kaposi's sarcoma

Aetiology and pathology

Kaposi's sarcoma has become increasingly common as a feature of the acquired immune deficiency syndrome (AIDS) or as a complication of deep immunosuppression. In these conditions Kaposi's sarcoma frequently appears in the mouth as a purplish plaque or nodule.

The tumour is thought to be of viral origin (possibly cytomegalovirus or HTLV III), either directly, or secondary to the immunodeficiency state.

Microscopy

Kaposi's sarcoma is a tumour of endothelial cells (as shown by the presence of factor VIII) but these largely assume a spindle shape. Early lesions consist of proliferating capillaries, usually with many inflammatory cells, and closely resemble granulation tissue.

Later there are fibrosarcoma-like interlacing bands of spindle-shaped tumour cells surrounding slit-like vessel lumens or minute round lumens when cut in cross-section. The inflammatory element progressively disappears, the tumour cells become more pleomorphic and mitoses become numerous. Interspersed are haemangioma-like areas with more obvious vascular spaces.

Kaposi's sarcoma has a poor prognosis in AIDS and is the cause of death in about 40% of these patients, usually within 2 or 3 years of diagnosis, irrespective of treatment.

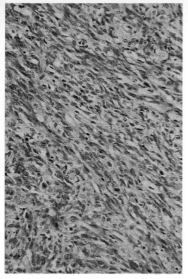

Fig. 203 Kaposi's sarcoma.

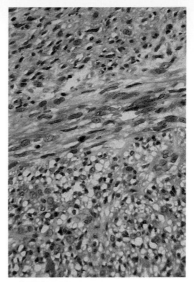

Fig. 204 Kaposi's sarcoma: spindle cells and transversely cut vascular spaces.

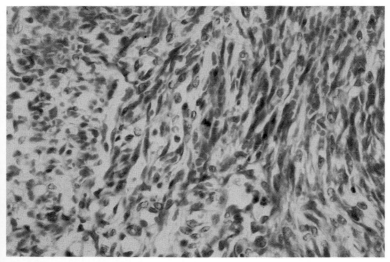

Fig. 205 Kaposi's sarcoma: mitotic activity.

Fibrosarcoma

Microscopy

Malignant fibroblasts form dense interlacing bundles of uniform, elongated, spindle-shaped cells with occasional mitoses and some collagen formation. With increasing dedifferentiation the arrangement of the cells becomes more irregular, mitoses become more frequent and less collagen is produced. Metastases may develop many years after diagnosis and usually in the lungs.

Rhabdomyosarcoma

Microscopy

The embryonal type consists of sheets of pleomorphic cells including tadpole-shaped rhabdomyoblasts. Cross-striation may be detectable.
In alveolar cell rhabdomyoscarcoma the tumour cells hang from the walls of slit-like (pseudoglandular) spaces and also form solid sheets.

Rhabdomyoma

Microscopy

Large, round, granular eosinophilic cells contain large amounts of glycogen and, frequently, fat spaces. Cross-striations may be found only with special staining.

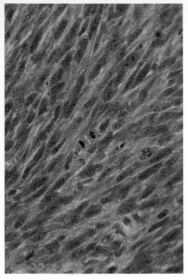

Fig. 206 Fibrosarcoma.

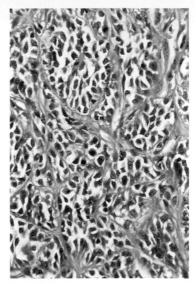

Fig. 207 Rhabdomyosarcoma: alveolar cell type.

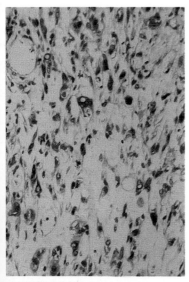

Fig. 208 Rhabdomyosarcoma: pleomorphic type.

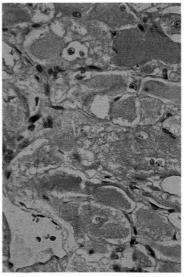

Fig. 209 Rhabdomyoma of tongue.

19 | Lymphomas

Lymphomas comprise Hodgkin's disease and non-Hodgkin's lymphoma. Non-Hodgkin's lymphoma usually arises from B lymphocytes and the different variants result from the stage of development of the lymphocyte undergoing neoplastic change. The cell of origin of Hodgkin's disease is uncertain but may be the monocyte or T lymphocyte.

Lymphomas (particularly Hodgkin's disease) are rare in the mouth and far more commonly affect cervical lymph nodes. In the mouth they may be the primary lesion or the presenting feature of disseminated disease.

Microscopy

Lymphomas are one of the most difficult areas of histopathology, as reflected by the many classifications. The essential feature is proliferation of lymphocytes either diffusely or with a follicular pattern. According to the type, the lumphocytes range from large immature lymphoblasts to small mature cells. Monoclonal immunoglobulin production may be detected. Surrounding tissues may be invaded. Hodgkin's disease is remarkable for the variety of cells present, including lymphocytes, histiocytes, eosinophils and Reed-Sternberg cells. The latter are large cells with a symmetrical (mirror-image) pair of large vesiculated nuclei.

The prognosis of non-Hodgkin's lymphoma varies according to the histological type and particularly to the stage of development when detected. Hodgkin's disease if reasonably localised responds to radiotherapy and/or chemotherapy.

ORAL PATHOLOGY

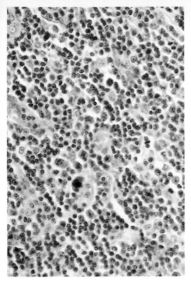

Fig. 210 Lymphocytic lymphoma.

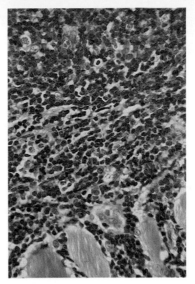

Fig. 211 Lymphoma invading muscle.

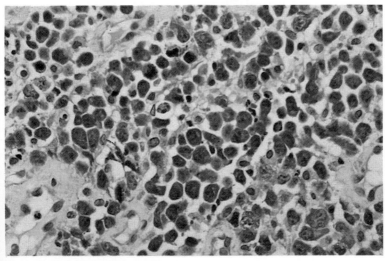

Fig. 212 Immunoblastic lymphoma.

Pigmented naevi

The pigment cells (melanocytes) can be intradermal (in the submucosal connective tissue), or junctional (the naevus cells cross the junction between the corium and the basal cells of the epithelium), appearing to drop down from the epithelium. In adults junctional activity is suggestive of development of malignant melanoma. Compound naevi show a combination of both features.

Malignant melanoma

Oral malignant melanomas are rare and are often large before being noticed.

Microscopy

The features can include (1) intraepithelial melanocytes, typically with clear halos round them, (2) junctional activity with melanocytes in large, clear areas within and dropping from the basal layer, (3) proliferation of melanocytes in the submucosal connective tissue. Malignant melanocytes range in shape from round to spindle-shaped and can be in solid sheets, rounded, circumscribed groups or in fascicles. Pigment may be dense or be invisible without special staining.

Amalgam tattoo

Clinically amalgam tattoos are by far the most common oral pigmented lesions. Histologically, the amalgam is seen as black particles or larger masses lying in the connective tissue and only rarely provokes a foreign body reaction. Biopsy may be needed to distinguish a tattoo from a pigmented tumour.

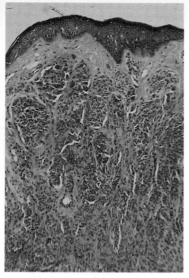

Fig. 213 Melanotic naevus.

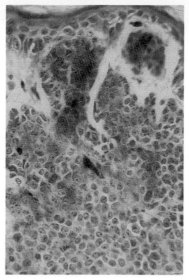

Fig. 214 Junctional activity and pigmentation.

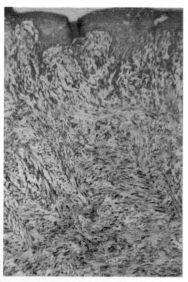

Fig. 215 Malignant melanoma: pigmented spindle-shaped melanocytes.

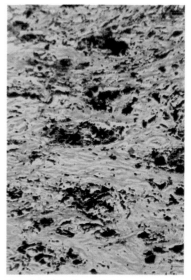

Fig. 216 Amalgam tattoo.

Miscellaneous Tumour-like Lesions

Granular cell myoblastoma

This is not regarded as a true tumour or as arising from myoblasts. The cell of origin is uncertain, but may be neural.

Microscopy

The two characteristic features are pseudo-epitheliomatous hyperplasia and granular cells. The overlying epithelium can closely mimic carcinoma, though it lacks cellular dysplasia. The granular cells are large and eosinophilic, and appear to be arising from degenerating muscle fibres.
It is benign and responds to excision.

Granular cell epulis of the newborn
(congenital epulis)

This rare epulis arises from the alveolar ridge in the newborn and consists of granular cells with well-defined cell membranes like those of granular cell myoblastoma but without intervening muscle fibres. The overlying epithelium is flat and pseudo-epitheliomatous hyperplasia is absent.

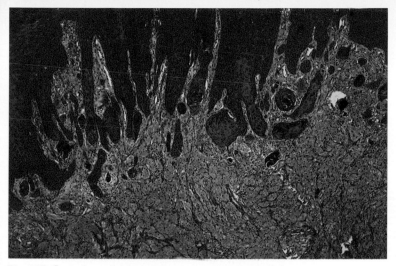

Fig. 217 Granular cell myoblastoma: pseudo-epitheliomatous hyperplasia.

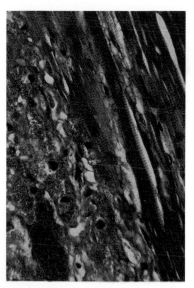

Fig. 218 Granular cell myoblastoma: muscle fibres and granular cells.

Pleomorphic adenoma

This is the most common type of salivary tumour but forms only about 40% of intra-oral salivary gland tumours. Typical sites are palate, lip and buccal glands.

Microscopy

Highly variable patterns are formed even within individual tumours. Common features include
1. duct-like structures
2. sheets of small, dark epithelial cells
3. squamous metaplasia and keratin formation
4. basophilic mucoid areas, sometimes forming the bulk of the tumour
5. cartilage and, occasionally, bone
6. fibroblast-like spindle cells
7. 'plasmacytoid' hyaline cells.

Pleomorphic adenomas are epithelial and the connective tissue structures are thought to result from activity of myoepithelial cells which have features in common with connective tissue cells. Myoepithelial cells cannot be identified with certainty by light microscopy, but probably form an important component of pleomorphic adenomas (spindle and hyaline cells for example).

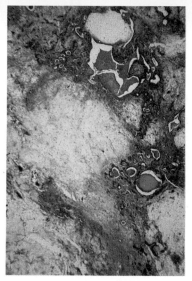

Fig. 219 Pleomorphic adenoma: typical mixed pattern.

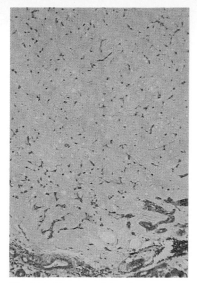

Fig. 220 Pleomorphic adenoma: myxomatous area.

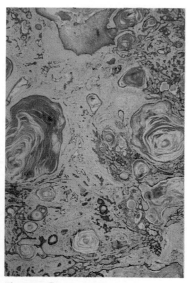

Fig. 221 Pleomorphic adenoma: squamous metaplasia.

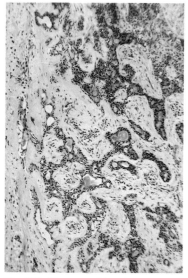

Fig. 222 Pleomorphic adenoma: tubular structures.

Pleomorphic adenoma (cont)

There is a fibrous capsule, but the tumour often extends through the capsule without invading surrounding tissues.

The tumour is slow-growing and benign but can undergo malignant change (carcinoma in pleomorphic adenoma) typically after many years of growth.

Complete excision is curative.

The tumour may also have an inductive effect on the stroma to produce the various connective tissue structures. Recurrence of pleomorphic adenomas results from

1. Surgical difficulties of removal, especially from the parotid.
2. Extension of tumour through the capsule.
3. Seeding of spilt tumour cells into the incision (attempted enucleation), leading to multinodular recurrences. (Pleomorphic adenomas are *not* initially multinodular.)

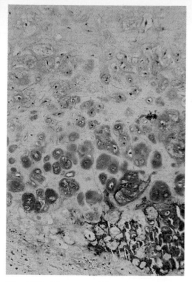

Fig. 223 Pleomorphic adenoma: cartilage with calcification.

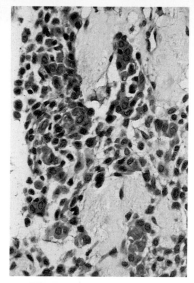

Fig. 224 Pleomorphic adenoma: hyaline cells.

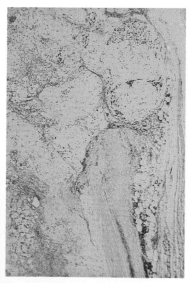

Fig. 225 Pleomorphic adenoma bulging through capsule.

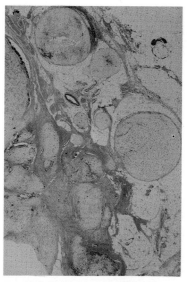

Fig. 226 Pleomorphic adenoma: multinodular recurrences.

Monomorphic adenomas

These have a uniform pattern often of trabecular or ductular pattern and lack the connective tissue components of pleomorphic adenoma. There are several subtypes.

Adenolymphoma (Warthin's tumour)

Adenolymphomas form about 10% of salivary gland tumours but virtually all are in the parotid and about 5% are bilateral. Intra-oral glands are probably never affected. This tumour is mostly seen in middle-age and typically forms a soft or cyst-like mass in the lower pole of the parotid.

Microscopy

The two components are glandular epithelium and lymphoid tissue. Tall, columnar, eosinophilic epithelial cells surround and protrude into cystic spaces and cover lymphoid tissue consisting of small lyphocytes and, usually, germinal centres. The tumour is benign.

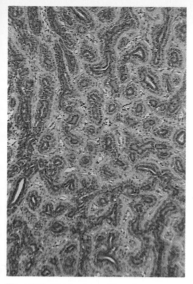

Fig. 227 Monomorphic adenoma.

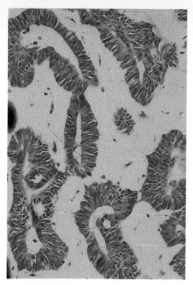

Fig. 228 Tubular monomorphic adenoma of lip.

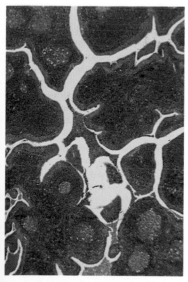

Fig. 229 Adenolymphoma.

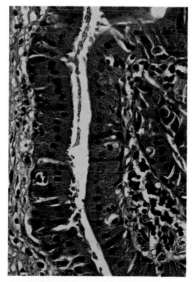

Fig. 230 Adenolymphoma: epithelial component.

Mucoepidermoid tumour

Mucoepidermoid tumour is relatively benign in most cases but can occasionally behave like a carcinoma. Forms nearly 10% of intra-oral salivary gland tumours; most commonly on the palate. Patients are usually middle-aged or older.

Microscopy

The two components are large, pale, mucus-secreting cells, which typically surround large or small cystic spaces, and sheets of epidermoid cells. Less well-differentiated tumours tend to resemble squamous cell carcinomas but for the presence of occasional mucous cells.
Behaviour is not reliably related to microscopic appearances. Wide excision is required.

Acinic cell tumour

Forms only about 2% of intra-oral salivary gland tumours.

Microscopy

Typically a more or less uniform pattern of large, darkly basophilic cells with granular cytoplasm, resembling serous acinar cells. Often tumour cells are in sheets without obvious organisation but occasionally in an acinar arrangement. Wide excision should be curative, and most malignant variants are rare.

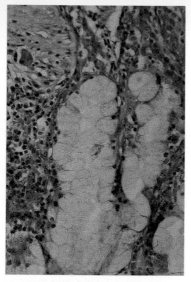

Fig. 231 Mucoepidermoid tumour.

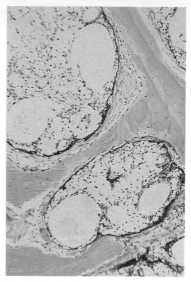

Fig. 232 Mucoepidermoid tumour invading bone.

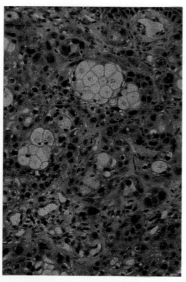

Fig. 233 Mucoepidermoid carcinoma.

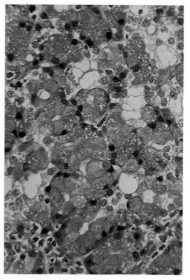

Fig. 234 Acinic cell tumour.

Adenoid cystic carcinoma

Forms 13% of intra-oral salivary gland tumours.

Microscopy

Consists of small, dark cells with duct-like 'holes' in a cribriform (Swiss cheese) or lace-like pattern, often with hyaline or mucinous change in the stroma. Strong tendency to perineural invasion and spread. The tumour is slow growing but difficult to excise as the borders are ill-defined. Metastases develop late and radical excision is needed.

Adenocarcinoma and other carcinomas

Form about 12% of intra-oral salivary gland tumours, and mainly affect the over 60s.

Microscopy

Well-differentiated tumours form glandular pattern or cysts with papillary ingrowths. Less well differentiated tumours show greater cellular pleomorphism.
Undifferentiated carcinomas and squamous cell carcinomas are rare and seen mostly in the elderly.

Carcinoma in pleomorphic adenoma

Pleomorphic adenoma can undergo malignant change, usually after years of slow growth. Carcinoma in pleomorphic adenoma comprises about 7% of salivary tumours of minor glands but up to 30% of sublingual gland tumours.

Microscopy

Malignant change is usually adenocarcinoma or undifferentiated carcinoma with invasion and destruction of surrounding structures, but elsewhere features of original pleomorphic adenoma persist.

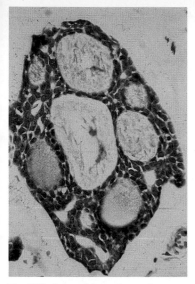

Fig. 235 Adenoid cystic carcinoma.

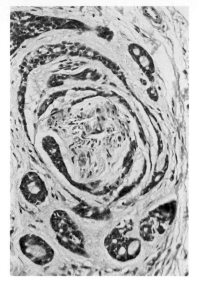

Fig. 236 Adenoid cystic carcinoma: perineural invasion.

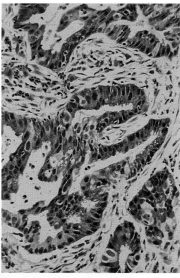

Fig. 237 Adenocarcinoma.

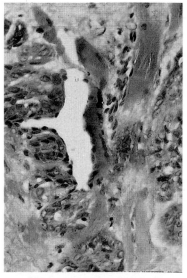

Fig. 238 Carcinoma in pleomorphic adenoma: muscle invasion.

23 | Salivary Gland Cysts

Mucous extravasation cysts (mucoceles)

Most common type of soft tissue cysts. Minor glands, especially of lip, affected.

Probably mainly result from injury to duct leading to leakage and formation of pools of saliva in overlying soft tissues with inflammatory reaction. Coalescence of pools of saliva leads to formation of cyst with lining of fibroblasts and compressed fibrous tissue.

Salivary retention cysts

Rare variant of mucocele produced by duct obstruction, forming a clinically similar lesion but cyst lined by flatted duct epithelium.

24 | Chronic Non-specific Sialadenitis (1)

Commonly a consequence of obstruction to salivary secretion, sometimes in association with calculus formation. Scattered, mainly periductal infiltration with chronic inflammatory cells, dilatation of ducts, degeneration of acini and increasing fibrous replacement (see Fig. 243).

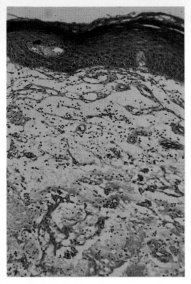

Fig. 239 Extravasation mucocele: early stage.

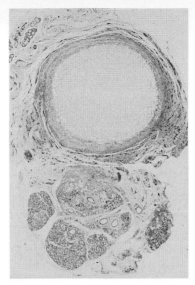

Fig. 240 Extravasation mucocele and attached salivary tissue.

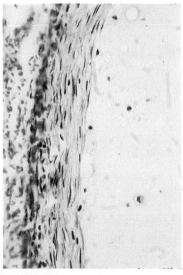

Fig. 241 Extravasation mucocele: fibrous wall.

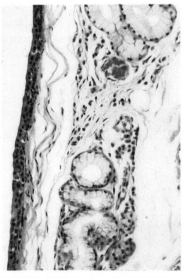

Fig. 242 Salivary mucous retention cyst: epithelial lining.

Salivary calculi

Calculi form usually by concretion of calcium salts round a nidus of organic matter, particularly in the submandibular gland. Calculi may be multiple within the gland or solitary and in the duct. Sialadenitis with duct dilatation is typically associated.

Calculi appear either as lamellated structures or multiple concretions which fuse to form a single mass. The surrounding duct epithelium may undergo squamous metaplasia and the surrounding tissue may be inflamed.

Sjögren's syndrome and related disorders

Sjögren's syndrome comprises dry mouth, dry eyes and connective tissue disease—usually rheumatoid arthritis. Sicca syndrome has no associated connective tissue disease and differs in the immunological findings. Benign lymphoepithelial lesion is the same histologically as Sjögren's syndrome. Mainly affect women, usually over 50.

Microscopy

Infiltration of salivary tissue by lymphocytes and plasma cells is initially periductal. Infiltrate spreads outwards and leads to progressive destruction of acini until only mononuclear cells and islands of hyperplastic duct epithelium ('epimyoepithelial islands') remain.

Lymphoplasmacytic infiltrate remains confined within the salivary lobules and does not penetrate the gland septa.

Labial salivary glands show close correlation with the parotid changes but epimyoepithelial islands rare.

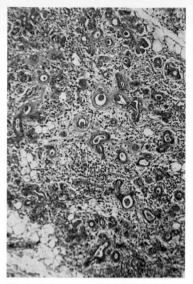

Fig. 243 Non-specific sialadenitis.

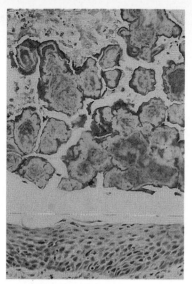

Fig. 244 Salivary calculi: squamous metaplasia of duct lining.

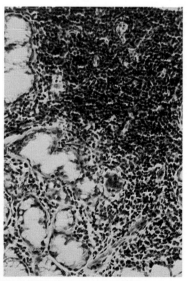

Fig. 245 Sjögren's syndrome: early stage.

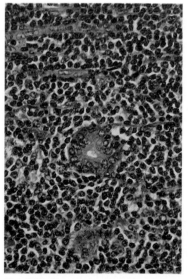

Fig. 246 Sjögren's syndrome: total destruction of gland acini.

Granulomatous Diseases (1)

Histologically, granulomas are focal, rounded collections of histiocytes, often with giant cells as in tuberculosis. Clinically however, 'granuloma' includes many chronic inflammatory conditions (e.g. apical granuloma, Wegener's granuloma, etc.) which lack granulomas histologically.

Tuberculosis

Aetiology

Typically secondary to long-standing pulmonary infection.

Microscopy

Deep ulcer with overhanging edges (usually on dorsum of tongue) with tuberculous granulomas and Langhan's giant cells.

Fungal infections (deep mycoses)

Immunosuppressed and AIDS patients are susceptible to many fungal infections such as histoplasmosis or aspergillosis. Other such infections are common in South America. Many produce oral lesions at some stage.

Microscopy

Many of the mycoses (*not* candidosis) produce granulomatous reactions more or less resembling tuberculosis. Tissue forms of the fungi may sometimes be detectable with special stains.

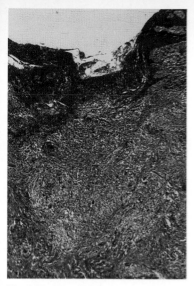

Fig. 247 Tuberculous ulcer of lip.

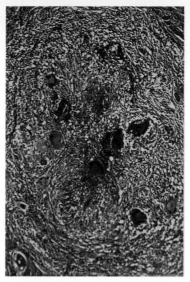

Fig. 248 Tuberculous granuloma beneath ulcer.

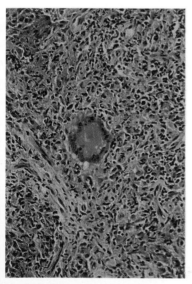

Fig. 249 Histoplasmosis of the tongue. Langhans giant cell and granuloma.

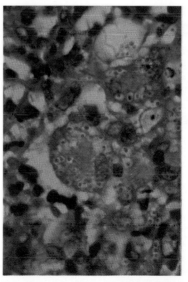

Fig. 250 *Histoplasma capsulatum:* spores surrounded by halo-like capsule.

Actinomycosis

Neither a mycosis nor a granulomatous disease histologically.

Microscopy

Actinomyces israelii from normal oral flora, if it invades the tissues, produces multiple abscesses. Suppuration with a central colony of this filamentous bacterium, surrounding fibrosis and sinuses develop.

Sarcoidosis

Aetiology

Unknown. Minor immunological defects— especially negative reaction to tuberculin.

Pathology

Hilar lymph nodes and sometimes peripheral lung are the main sites but almost any tissue can be affected. Predilection also for salivary tissue, especially labial glands. Gingival enlargement in some cases.

Microscopy

Compact histiocytic granulomas without caseation, often multiple and with dense lymphocytic infiltrate.

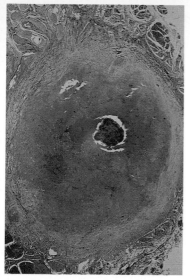

Fig. 251 Actinomycosis: loculus with central colony surrounded by neutrophils and fibrous abscess wall.

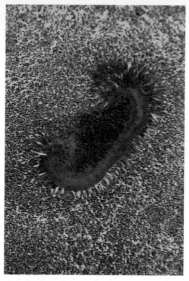

Fig. 252 Actinomycosis: detail of bacterial colony.

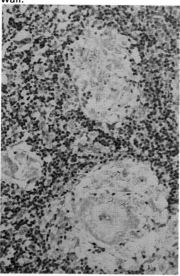

Fig. 253 Sarcoidosis: typical granuloma with giant cell.

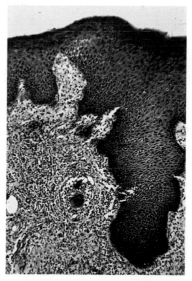

Fig. 254 Crohn's disease of oral mucosa (see p. 139).

Crohn's disease

Aetiology unknown. Typically causes granulomatous inflammation of ileum but can involve many other sites including the mouth. Oral lesions include cobblestone proliferation of mucosa and sometimes ulceration.

Microscopy

Subepithelial oedema, minor chronic inflammation and usually small, loose scattered granulomas either superficially or deeply. *Note.* Melkersson Rosenthal syndrome (facial or labial swelling, recurrent facial palsies and fissured tongue) and cheilitis granulomatosa show similar histology.

Midline granulomas

A diverse group of diseases characterised by facial or nasopharyngeal inflammation or necrosis and usually involvement of lungs or kidneys. Not related to granulomas described above. Oral lesions develop in some variants, especially Wegener's granulomatosis.

Wegener's granulomatosis
Comprises chronic necrotising inflammation of upper respiratory tract, vasculitis associated with giant cells and glomerulonephritis. Occasionally a characteristic florid chronic proliferative gingivitis ('strawberry' gums) with giant cells.

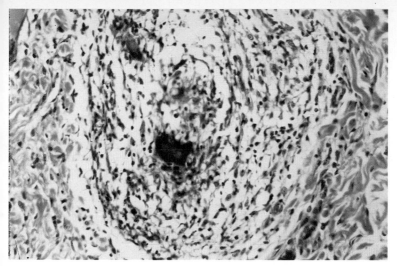

Fig. 255 Crohn's disease: granuloma in oral connective tissue.

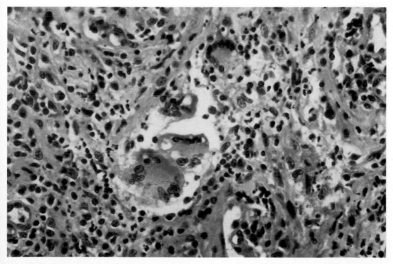

Fig. 256 Wegener's granulomatosis: typical giant cells in gingival biopsy.

Progressive systemic sclerosis
(scleroderma)

A connective tissue (autoimmune) disease producing progressive fibrosis and stiffening of the skin and viscera. Limitation of opening and movement of the tongue and Sjögren's syndrome may develop. Antinuclear bodies present. Death usually from renal or cardiac failure.

Microscopy

Progressive fibrous thickening of submucosa extending into and destroying superficial muscle fibres. Perivascular lymphocytic infiltrate.

Oral submucous fibrosis

Affects those from Indian subcontinent but aetiology unknown: not autoimmune. Intense symmetrical board-like thick stiffening of sites such as palate, cheeks or lip but not viscera or other parts of the body.

Microscopy

Similar to scleroderma but more intense and lacking perivascular infiltrate. Sometimes epithelial dysplasia—possibly premalignant.

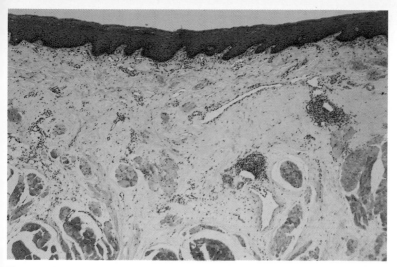

Fig. 257 Scleroderma: submucosal fibrosis with muscle destruction in the tongue and perivascular lymphocytic infiltrate.

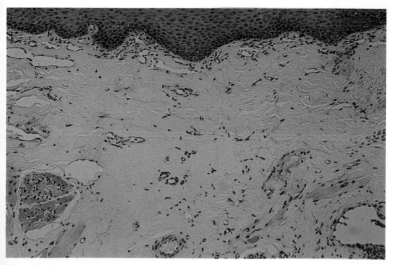

Fig. 258 Oral submucous fibrosis: Deeper extension of fibrosis and muscle destruction than in scleroderma.

CHURCHILL LIVINGSTONE
Medical Division of Longman Group UK Limited

Distributed in the United States of America by Churchill Livingstone Inc.,
1560 Broadway, New York, N.Y. 10036, and by associated companies,
branches and representatives throughout the world.

First published 1987

ISBN 0 — 443 — 03142 — 8

British Library Cataloguing in Publication Data

Cawson, R.A.
    Oral pathology.—(Colour aids)
    1. Teeth—Diseases   2. Mouth—Diseases
    I. Title   II. Series
    617'.52207   RK307

Library of Congress Cataloging in Publication Data

Cawson, R.A.
    Oral pathology.
    (Colour aids)
    1. Mouth—Diseases—Atlases. I. Title. II. Series.
[DNLM: 1. Dentistry—atlases. 2. Jaw Diseases—
atlases. 3. Mouth Diseases—atlases. WU 17 C3830]
RC815.C394 1987   617'.522   86–9723

Produced by Longman Group (FE) Ltd
Printed in Hong Kong.